"A straightforward and commonsensical glide path into fine-tuning one of the most fundamental relationships in our lives, namely with food, for the sake of well-being, health, happiness, and social connection. This book will nourish and support you in multiple ways and, if you stick with its recommendations for practicing mindfulness, will give you more than a taste of who is eating in the first place, and why."

—**Jon Kabat-Zinn**, author of *Mindfulness for Beginners*

"Lynn Rossy takes us on a most uplifting and exquisite journey. She shows us how by bringing more consciousness to our eating, we can truly nourish ourselves and experience genuine well-being. She shows us how to have a healthy relationship with our bodies and minds, understand our habits while not being run by them, learn to listen to the wisdom right inside of us, and discover how to truly savor life. Clear, practical, and engaging, *The Mindfulness-Based Eating Solution* makes the process of taking good care of ourselves inspiring and fun. A wonderful book!"

—**James Baraz**, coauthor of *Awakening Joy*, and cofounding teacher at Spirit Rock Meditation Center in Woodacre, CA

"*The Mindfulness-Based Eating Solution* gives anyone who has struggled with food a realistic and achievable approach to finding peace with food and eating. While founded on solid science, Lynn Rossy offers a supportive, nurturing, and real-life approach to inviting change while still enjoying the foods you love. *The Mindfulness-Based Eating Solution* will have you savoring each bite, appreciating your body, and leaving each meal feeling satisfied. Why beat up on yourself and continue to eat on autopilot? This excellent book gives you a clear road map for getting off the diet merry-go-round and building a healthy relationship to food!"

—**Donald Altman, MA, LPC**, author of
The Mindfulness Toolbox, Clearing Emotional Clutter, and *12-Weeks to Mindful Eating*

"Reading this book is like talking to a wise and warmhearted friend—a friend who has the knowledge and experience to help you reclaim the natural pleasure and daily satisfaction that is inherent in eating. As an added bonus, it's filled with helpful exercises and tips based on scientific studies, including the author's own research."

—**Jan Chozen Bays, MD**, author of *Mindful Eating*

The
Mindfulness-Based
Eating
Solution

proven strategies to

end overeating, satisfy your

hunger & savor your life

Lynn Rossy, PhD

New Harbinger Publications, Inc.

Publisher's Note

This publication is designed to provide accurate and authoritative information in regard to the subject matter covered. It is sold with the understanding that the publisher is not engaged in rendering psychological, financial, legal, or other professional services. If expert assistance or counseling is needed, the services of a competent professional should be sought.

Distributed in Canada by Raincoast Books

Copyright © 2016 by Lynn Rossy
New Harbinger Publications, Inc.
5674 Shattuck Avenue
Oakland, CA 94609
www.newharbinger.com

Cover design by Amy Shoup
Acquired by Jess O'Brien
Edited by Rona Bernstein

Library of Congress Cataloging-in-Publication Data on file

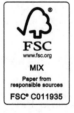 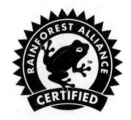

18   17   16

10   9   8   7   6   5   4   3   2   1   First Printing

To Ginny Morgan, who introduced me to the practice of mindfulness. Her gentle, wise spirit has surely helped me write this book, even from the heavenly realms.

Contents

Introduction

If you have ever struggled with how to eat or felt dissatisfied with your body, this book is for you. These two interrelated issues can cause tremendous emotional distress, guilt, shame, depression, and anxiety. Instead of inspiring healthy behavior, efforts to change often result in unhealthy weight-control strategies, binge eating, reduced physical activity, and poorer overall health.

No matter how old you are, what you look like, or what number appears on the scale, the battle with food and the destructive criticism of our bodies is epidemic in size and scale. This phenomenon holds true for women and men, although women are known to report it more often. Almost everybody would like to have a better relationship with food and their bodies.

The culture we live in and the environments we work in compound our troubles. The conditions of the modern workplace—offices filled with unhealthy food choices and jobs that often require sitting for hours in front of a computer—make it extremely difficult to nourish our bodies with the right food and regular movement. Whether we work in an office or not, our culture compels us to be busy, overworked, overscheduled, and distracted—conditions which do not support making good choices for our physical, mental, and emotional well-being. Combine these circumstances with the constant barrage of conflicting information and advertisements telling us the perfect way to eat and look, and you have a recipe for discontent and dysfunction.

Although the difficulties people face as they seek a better relationship with food and their bodies are extremely complex and varied, there is an underlying thread that ties them together. That thread is the very natural longing of body, mind, and heart for greater health and well-being. That longing brought you to this book.

As a health psychologist at a university wellness program, I was given the task of developing a program to help people overcome their issues with weight. Being a heterogeneous community, we needed something that would appeal to people who fall along the continuum of underweight to overweight. I brought my own past experiences with binge eating and being overweight, my personal and professional practice of mindfulness, and my true love of food to the task. What developed was a holistic approach to weight management that included a broad view of health. When you start to become healthy with regard to food, you simultaneously become a healthier person in all aspects of your life.

Witnessing the restoration to a healthy mind and body experienced by people when they use the concepts and ideas found in this book has been a great honor and joy. In fact, it has become my greatest passion. I hope you join these people in taking the same steps to restore your relationship to food and your body.

It can be helpful to have a notebook or journal to record your thoughts, feelings, and experiences as you read through the book. Writing can help you explore new information, reveal insights, and clarify your wisdom. It can provide a record of your understanding and growth about this new way of eating and living.

Throughout the book, I share the stories of people whose lives have been changed through the practices you find in each chapter. The stories are authentic, although the names of people have been changed to preserve privacy and confidentiality. On occasion, composite characters are used in order to condense common themes. You aren't alone and these stories prove it.

Writing this book has been an extremely satisfying labor of love. I have tried to flavor it with the excitement and enthusiasm I feel at the prospect of helping others through the words on these pages. It is my sincere wish that this book be a guide for you to having a life that's filled with the joys of eating, moving your body in ways that feel delicious, mastering the skills to overcome difficulties without using food, and embracing the fullness of the life you were meant to live.

CHAPTER 1

You Can Have Your Cake and Eat It Too!

How did *eating* get so complicated? There is an increasing amount of diet advice and plans available, and yet the prominent result has been to overwhelm and confuse people about how to nurture themselves. Our struggles with food have simultaneously created a war with our bodies. By using the practices in this book, you will be able to restore harmony with food and reunite with your body.

The search for a better way to eat might be motivated by a desire to weigh less, have more energy, look younger, and be healthier. Somehow if you can just "get it right"—which might mean seeing the right number on the scale or getting into the right pants size—you'll be okay. You've searched the marketplace for answers to your diet and health concerns, but your efforts to change have not been as successful or lasting as you'd like them to be. You might feel a fleeting sense of happiness or satisfaction when you lose a pound or two, but you either gain it back or decide it wasn't enough.

After feeling frustrated or defeated too many times, you might be saying, "Screw it, I'm going to eat whatever I want. I'll show you!" You overeat out of rebellion against restrictive diets, scolding parents, helpful advice, a "skinny is in" culture, or the little voice in your head telling you how you *should* eat. Of course, when you do rebel, you have to pay the price with the scolding you give yourself afterward and the weight that suddenly appears on your body.

If you haven't yet mastered how to eat and live with complete joy and ease, don't feel discouraged. Most road maps have taken you in the wrong direction—looking outside of yourself for answers, validation, satisfaction, and happiness. On one hand, you are told what diet to be on to restrict your food choices. On the other hand, you are driven by a culture that tells you consumption is correlated with happiness. You eat, drink, and shop as a way of feeding yourself what you think you need in order to feel okay or make you numb enough not to care.

It's not surprising if you find yourself in a position of having overconsumed. Millions of dollars are spent on advertising so that you seek and buy, but this definitely does not yield a real solution to your hunger—whether it's a hunger for food or a deeper hunger not fixed by filling up your belly. The search outside yourself to meet your needs is designed not to work.

Alternatively, the real joy of eating and living depends on a clear understanding of hunger, an awareness of what you're really hungry for, and the ability to satisfy your desires in a way that leads to health and well-being. The road map you will find in the pages of this book, first and foremost, is instruction in the skill of mindfulness and how to use it in the service of what you've been searching for—whether that's a slimmer body, more energy, or greater happiness.

Quite simply, mindfulness is about tuning in to the present moment with kindness and curiosity. Mindfulness not only helps you make better food choices, but also helps you bring a quality of kindness toward everything, including your body.

By mindfully encountering the present, you can learn to make better decisions in all areas of your life and develop a growing trust in your inner guidance. You will become aware of body sensations, thoughts, and feelings you've never noticed before. This information provides the inner guideposts for making the decisions that nourish and enrich you.

The practice of mindfulness is the opposite of the practice of judgment and gives you a much needed break from a pretty pathological belief that we need to be flawless. Relating to yourself and your body in a more positive way means you not only feel better but end up treating yourself better as well. Healthier decisions flow from a kind view of oneself. As hard as it might be to grasp just yet, the more you accept yourself, just as you are, the easier it will be to act in ways that lead you to greater health.

In this chapter, I'll present an approach that teaches you how to eat when you're hungry and not eat more than you need, while savoring and enjoying each bite. In other words, you CAN have your cake and eat it too, with great delight! You will be encouraged to take a few beginning steps to start a journey of discovery that ends the struggles you have with food, your body, and maybe even your life.

You can start by asking yourself the question *What am I hungry for?* As you learn to explore this question, you will quickly discover that the answer isn't always food, but hungers as diverse as the need for support, friendship, movement, silence, fun, reflection, work, play, rest, romance, nature, and creativity. In essence, by discovering what you are truly hungry for, you might find your life being guided in ways you've never imagined.

Don't worry. You don't have to move to a new city, find a new job, or divorce your spouse. However, if your life needs some fine-tuning, mindfulness will certainly be a useful guide. Looking at your current life through the lens of mindfulness creates the conditions for a new way of relating to your life. In fact, if you haven't heard of mindfulness until now, consider the possibility that you have all of the answers you need, but you just haven't noticed.

THE MINDFULNESS-BASED EATING SOLUTION

Throughout the rest of this chapter, I will describe the foundational components of a mindfulness-based intuitive eating program called Eat for Life that inspired this book. You will learn about the research demonstrating its success and read testimonials from people who have used this program that powerfully attest to its impact in their lives. We'll have a frank talk about diets and why it's important to give them up while you're learning to investigate your inner signals about how to eat. Finally, I'll suggest a few steps to help you get started with this non-diet approach to weight management and eating with the greatest pleasure.

Mindfulness

The first feature of the program is mindfulness. Because the key to making the changes you want requires looking inside yourself for your answers, practicing mindfulness is essential. Mindfulness is the ultimate guide and ally in helping you make better food choices. Beyond self-discipline or willpower, it's about the power of awareness. Behavior change happens when you become aware of what you're doing and why you're doing it.

Decades of research have demonstrated the impact of mindfulness. At the risk of making it sound like a panacea, research has shown that people who practice mindfulness experience significant physical improvements in weight, sleep, pain, and immune system functioning (Grossman et al. 2004) as well as psychological improvements in stress, anxiety, depression, behavioral regulation, and emotional reactivity (Keng, Smoski, and Robins 2011). Truly, most of the issues that challenge us can be unraveled and improved with mindfulness.

Intuitive Eating

The second feature of the program is intuitive eating. The principles of intuitive eating guide you to follow your internal signals, such as physical hunger and satiety cues, when determining how to eat—instead of reaching for food when something upsets you or just when food is there. Intuitive eating has emerged as a promising alternative to restrictive dieting based on external rules and stimuli such as rigid meal times and calorie counts (Gast and Hawks 2000;

Tribole and Resch 1995). The three components of intuitive eating are (a) granting oneself unconditional permission to eat when and what the body desires, (b) eating in response to physical versus emotional cues, and (c) relying on internal cues of hunger and satiety to evaluate what, when, and how much to eat (Tylka 2006).

Research has demonstrated that people with higher scores on an intuitive eating scale are significantly more likely to have better physical health (e.g., lower body mass index, better blood lipid profiles, and lower cardiovascular risk; Hawks et al. 2005) and greater psychological well-being (e.g., lower self-consciousness and higher pleasure from eating; Smith and Hawks 2006). Additionally, higher scores on intuitive eating are associated with less disordered eating behavior.

Mindless Eating

The third feature of the program is awareness of how you mindlessly eat. You might be thinking you don't need any extra instruction in how to eat mindlessly! But, the key is how to be more aware of it. We live in a world that supports and encourages mindless eating, resulting in increased consumption and eating food that isn't very healthy. In his book *Mindless Eating,* Brian Wansink (2006) describes marketing research and highlights the many ways we get tricked into eating more than we think we need (e.g., portion sizes, large plates and bowls, distraction, labeling). An illumination of when you mindlessly eat will support your efforts to eat more mindfully.

AND THE RESEARCH SAYS...

After teaching the Eat for Life program for a couple of years, I decided to put it to the test of scientific examination. I worked with a wonderful graduate student, Hannah Bush, who undertook this project for her doctoral dissertation. We compared one group of women who went through the Eat for Life program to another group of women who did not go through the program. At the end of ten weeks, the women in the Eat for Life group were significantly more successful at eating in response to their bodily cues (intuitive eating), more appreciative of their bodies, less likely to binge eat, and more mindful. Further, the practice of mindfulness was, as I suspected, a significant reason for all of the other positive changes the women experienced (Bush et al. 2014). (Note to men: Several men went through the program as well, but we did not include them in the study because they were significantly fewer in number. They definitely benefitted along with the women.)

The same benefits can be yours. If you're tired of the tyranny and eventual failure of the next new diet, frustrated with your weight, unhappy with your body, or simply trying to figure out how to eat more healthily, now is the time to take back your life. Perhaps you eat when you're stressed, unhappy, happy, restless, frustrated, or bored. Perhaps you eat mindlessly in front of the computer and the TV. Perhaps you eat because food is cheap, fast, and easy. No matter what your individual story entails, you can sit down with this book and discover a way to end the struggle and make a lasting truce with food, your body, and your life.

AND THE PARTICIPANTS SAY...

After going through the program, participants report many changes, but a few themes emerge that demonstrate the dramatic shift in the ability to nourish and nurture oneself. I've condensed them into three statements: *I love the food I eat*; *I feel good after eating the food I love*; *I respect and care for my body*.

Love the food you eat. Are you loving and savoring the food you eat? If your answer is often no, there are plenty of reasons why you're not getting the most out of your eating experiences. For starters, you may not really be paying attention to how your food tastes. You might think you like the food you're eating, but prepare yourself to be surprised. As you learn to be present with curiosity and interest when you eat and drink, more and more subtle flavors and tastes will be revealed. Regularly people tell stories of being amazed when they notice, for the first time, how some favorite food they thought they enjoyed actually tastes like chemicals, artificial flavors, or just not like food.

Karen is a prime example. After practicing mindful eating for two weeks, she exclaimed, "I don't like anything I eat. But, I just hadn't ever noticed before!" That statement really blew me over and demonstrates how unconscious we can be about food. Karen eventually discovered the food she loved to eat. She also came face to face with other things she hadn't noticed about her life. The path of rediscovering your taste and the pleasure of food can lead to the discovery of other new and tastier ways to lead your entire life.

Another obstacle to loving your food is feeling guilty about eating the food you love. Guilt, unlike regret, is an emotion that shuts you down and often gives rise to shame. Guilt frequently leads to eating food in secret, eating too much, and eating the food you love but getting no pleasure out of it. So eat (without guilt) the food you find yummy and take time to enjoy the experience of eating. If you eat too much of it you might feel regret, which can be a powerful motivator for change, but don't feel guilty for having eaten it in the first place.

"*Savor your food* is the most powerful teaching I've learned. Sitting with each bite and just giving in to enjoyment makes every food item and every meal a thing of joy. And moments of joy during the day are something worth cherishing." This testimony, written by Erica, speaks volumes about the adventure you're about to take. As Tribole and Resch (1995, 143) propose in their book, *Intuitive Eating*, "If you don't love it, don't eat it, and if you love it, savor it!"

Love the way you *feel* when you eat the food you love. You might be saying, "I love food and that's the problem." Loving food, in and of itself, is not a problem if you also love the way you *feel* after you eat it. When you consciously decide to eat food that makes you feel alive, gives you energy, and helps your body be healthy, you get to love your food and feel good at the same time. You might not know what that feels like yet, but when I eat this way, I can actually feel my belly smiling at me. I'll give you a hint: this doesn't happen after devouring a bag of French fries.

Kayla reported that after she consumes junk food, she feels very groggy. "I can't eat much of it before my body starts screaming, 'I need real food! I need vegetables! Give them to me now!'" She said, "When I eat what my body loves I feel really good about myself and how I feel, knowing it is exactly what my body needs."

Loving the way you *feel* after you eat the food you love also happens when you don't completely stuff yourself. You can have your cake and eat it too, but how much of a good thing is good? One of the most important discoveries you will make when you slow down and really savor your food (particularly the cake) is that you don't need nearly as much of it. Sometimes you'll even discover that cake isn't what you really wanted.

If you're skeptical, that's okay. You don't have to take my word for any of these ideas. The best thing about this book is you get to try out my suggestions and see for yourself. *You* will learn to be the expert about *your* body and what it needs and why.

Respect and care for your body. Barbara found the mindful eating concepts puzzling at first. She didn't see how allowing herself to eat the food she wanted, even if she was really mindful about it, wouldn't lead to overeating. Every week she reported that she would make a pan of brownies in the evening (this apparently happened a lot) and eat five or six of them in one sitting. In class, I'd go over all of the steps of mindful eating (including paying attention to the signal from your body that says "stop"), but she insisted this was not helping her with the brownie situation.

The turning point came when I introduced the idea of respecting your body. "What does it mean to respect your body?" I asked. Let's face it, unless you're a small child, you are the central person responsible for treating your body with respect, so it is a pretty important question to consider. Does the type and amount of food you put in your mouth show respect for your body?

Looking as if a light bulb had gone off in her head, Barbara exclaimed, "I get it! If I respected my body then I wouldn't put a pan of brownies in it in one sitting." This one moment of insight completely altered Barbara's paradigm around food and her body. The next time she made brownies, she ate only ONE! She discovered that to respect her body meant to feed it with respect, and it didn't need more than one.

Respect can be shown by how much we eat, but it can be shown in a variety of other ways as well. Throughout the book we'll be talking about how you can respect your body by moving and stretching it on a regular basis, by giving it the sleep it needs, and by talking to it with kind and caring words.

The respect you have for your body not only changes how you treat it, but ultimately translates into respect for other bodies around you—improving your relationships with others.

Natalie said, "I appreciate and respect my body. It has given birth to beautiful children, survived cancer and diabetes. It may not look like the ideal body, but it's mine and it has survived through thick and thin. Even the scars are beautiful to me, for they reaffirm that I'm alive." This is such a beautiful affirmation of life and being human. Now is your time to learn what it means to honor your worth as a human being.

OVERCOMING THE DIET MENTALITY

As I mentioned earlier, we need to talk about diets. This book espouses a non-diet approach to weight management that flies in the face of our conditioning. Dieting seems to be embedded in our culture to the point of being compulsory. Do you remember the time when you simply ate when you were hungry and didn't worry about calories, weight, health, or how you looked? If you're like me, that was many years ago. And, it's not our fault. There are many forces conspiring to keep us unhappy and dissatisfied with the way we look and the way we eat. One of the biggest forces is the hundreds of diets vying for our attention and our money.

Review your dieting history. How many have you been on? Are you on one now? The research I conducted revealed that participants were actively on a diet for an average of 39 percent of their lives—some starting their diets as young as five years old! And, the negative impact from this early indoctrination to dieting ranges from being overweight to feeling miserable about ourselves.

Diets Don't Work

It is easy to be attracted by promises of amazing results in thirty days, the diet that a friend is trying, or a claim that you'll be smarter, stronger, and happier with a particular product. You intuitively know the results you seek are going to take some time and effort, but you still hold out hope for the quick fix. The secret hope is you will melt down to your perfect shape or have a healthier body and it's all going to happen quickly and easily. But, let's be honest with each other. If any of the diets you've been on had been successful (however you define that), would you really be reading this book?

Diets, in particular, have done very little to help people lose weight or curb anyone's appetite. At least that's what the statistics say. America's obesity rates are among the highest in the world.

Millions of people are on diets, yet two thirds of US adults are over-weight or obese and these numbers and waistlines are continuing to grow (Ogden et al. 2014). There is a multibillion dollar global weight-loss industry banking on the fact that you'll need its diet products for a long time.

Researchers at the University of California, Los Angeles ana-lyzed the results from thirty-one long-term studies of diets and con-cluded that even if dieters lose weight initially, the majority of people on diets gain all of the weight back, plus more. "Yo-yo" dieters, people who lose and gain weight, especially repeatedly, actually increase their risks for diabetes, hypertension, heart disease, and metabolic syndrome (Mann et al. 2007). This review of the litera-ture demonstrates that you are actually better off never having gone on a diet in the first place.

Many diets are considered by clinicians and researchers to pose significant health risks and offer minimal long-term benefits. This is particularly true of "crash" or "fad" diets—short-term weight-loss plans that involve caloric or food restrictions and drastic changes to a person's normal eating habits. Someone on a strict calorie-restricted diet is sending messages to the body that she is starving, resulting in the body storing fat, which is in direct opposition to the desired effect. The take-home message is "diets don't work" (at least not for most people and not in the long term).

I've heard plenty of anecdotal evidence of dismal dieting fail-ures. Stacey, a long-term dieter, stated, "I have done so many diets since I was fifteen years old, I can tell you how many calories are in any kind of food." She went on to validate what the research tells us: "Diets never worked out. No matter what kind of diet plan I have ever tried, nothing was permanent. I would weigh myself constantly, and the weight always came back."

Like Stacey, many dieters are frustrated and have thrown up their hands in disgust. Paula said, "Because of my diet history, I have reached a point where I do not even feel capable of dieting. All the platitudes in the world cannot motivate me at this point. I have tried just about every diet possible and that is not a way for me to live. I am one of those people that hear the word 'diet' and immediately start eating everything in sight."

Even if you are someone who says you don't diet, you might be surprised at how influenced you are by the diet mentality. You say you aren't on a diet, but you secretly dread the times when your food options are not within your control, you examine food carefully before you eat it, you label foods as "good" and "bad," or you have a lot of shoulds and shouldn'ts when it comes to eating. You may say you just want to eat healthily, but you deny yourself the pleasure of eating if it doesn't fall into the "good" category. (Note: There is a difference between the diet mentality and mindfully deciding you don't want to eat certain foods after an examination of their taste and effect on your body.) Because of their omnipresence, dieting thoughts and images are ingrained in us all.

Take a moment right now and check in with yourself. Even though this book takes a clearly "non-diet" approach, you might unconsciously be hoping it's the next new diet plan that will actually work. Be honest with yourself. The "dieting mind" is very clever.

Why Diets Don't Work

So, why don't diets work? First, diets overly restrict the kinds of food or how much food you can eat, so you would never be able to continue to eat this way in the long term. Eating a limited variety of food or consuming deathly low calorie counts will help you lose weight while you're on the diet, but when you go off of it and start eating as you normally do (which you will), you gain the weight back. This is the yo-yo dieting I talked about earlier.

Second, research demonstrates that after a calorie-restricted diet, you not only will start eating as you did before, but will probably eat more. In the often-cited Minnesota Starvation Experiment, when participants were allowed to eat whatever they wanted after being restricted, they had insatiable appetites yet never felt full, and these effects continued for months afterward (Keys et al. 1950). Further, after six months of a "semi-starvation" diet (1560 calories), participants demonstrated marked depression, irritability, intense preoccupation with thoughts of food, a decrease in self-initiated activity, loss of sexual drive, and social introversion.

Third, what happens when you tell yourself you can't have something to eat? You want it! Right? And when you finally have it, you'll have a lot of it. Oftentimes you'll eat your forbidden food alone and in secret while no one is watching. You'll gobble it down as fast as you can so nobody sees you. You'll have to have a lot of it because you tell yourself you're never going to have it again.

My friend Lynn wouldn't allow herself to have candy and sweets at home, so she would steal those goodies from the desk drawers of her coworkers. Of course, it was kind of a joke because all of her coworkers knew she was doing it. They gladly stocked their drawers for her stealing pleasure. Janice, a twenty-five-year-old athlete, would only sneak cookies and sweets at work because her athletic husband tried to keep her on a very strict calorie and carb count. Both of these women were not going to be denied, but they didn't really get to enjoy their treats, indulging alone and in secret.

Fourth, when you're relying solely on an outside source (such as a diet) to tell you what to eat, you're not paying attention to the wisdom of your own body. Until you begin to listen to and trust your inner wisdom (instead of a diet) about what, when, why, and how much you eat, it is unlikely you will be able to change the way you eat. The body has amazing sensors for what food is healthy, what food is poison to the system, how much food it needs to consume, and what nutrition it needs. Animals in the wild live and eat by instinctive internal wisdom and forage the fields and forests for the food that will meet their nutritional requirements. No one had to give them a nutrition class, and yet they are very capable of knowing what to eat. We are no less intuitive than animals, but most humans have cut themselves off from the body's natural guidance.

This brings me to the last and maybe most important point: diets tend to take the joy out of food. On a diet, the only joy is found when you cheat—and you will! My philosophy is that food is a wonderful part of our lives, to be enjoyed and savored. A non-diet approach to weight management is one that celebrates the pleasure found in culinary delights of all kinds. When you truly savor your food, you are slowing down to taste the moment and the juiciness of life.

BEGINNING STEPS TO TAKE

Under your nose, in your belly, on your tongue, in your eyes, and in your mind you have the knowledge you need to be wisely instructed about what, when, why, and how much to eat. Instead of eating to fix or deny your feelings, you will learn to respond to difficult times with kindness and courage. You will uncover the thoughts and beliefs that keep sabotaging your efforts to eat better and be healthier so that YOU are in the driver's seat when you make decisions about how to eat and live. Along with the transformation in how you relate to food, you can discover an admiration for your body (no matter what size you are) that supports your efforts to take better care of it.

Before you go any farther, here are a few things I'd like you to consider that will help you turn your focus inward. This won't happen overnight, but these next steps will prepare you to dive into the rest of the program laid out in the book.

1. Get Off the Diets

If you aren't on one, great. If you are, experiment with not dieting during the time it takes you to read and work with the concepts in this book. Only by not dieting can you give yourself a chance to discover your internal sources of guidance.

However, if your doctor has you on a specific regimen for a medical issue, by all means continue on it. Everything I write about in this book can be modified to fit your needs. People with diabetes or who are prediabetic have found that the concepts in this book gave them the tools to be more successful with the directives from their doctor. The skills you learn will help you feel better about, succeed at, and enjoy the diet that you need to be on.

2. Get Off the Scale

My recommendation is to put the scale away *now* and don't weigh yourself again until you've read and worked with the exercises in the book (if ever again). Despite any slight to significant anxiety this creates for you, I hope you give yourself the opportunity to discover what staying off the scale can teach you. Not relying on an external measurement to monitor your weight helps you begin your journey inward. This is the first step toward listening to your internal signals to guide how you eat. Besides, you can gauge getting heavier or lighter by paying attention to how your body looks and feels or how tight or loose your pants fit.

Has getting on the scale ever helped you lose weight? Or are you ever happy with the number on the scale? I've asked these questions to many people and the answer is usually a resounding no. Getting off the scale lets you stop creating one time a day that you purposely feel disappointed with yourself.

Personally, my game with the scale was to set a weight that I wanted to but couldn't realistically meet. Years went by and then a miracle happened. I finally, and incredibly, reached my goal. I was so happy—for about two seconds (literally)—before I decided I needed to be five pounds lighter! A long time ago, I left the scale with my ex-husband, and I've been a lot happier ever since.

One issue that makes not weighing yourself difficult is a trip to the doctor, since the first thing you are asked to do is get on the scale. Having dealt with this for years, here is what I suggest: tell the nurse you will get on the scale but you don't want to know how much you weigh. Even if you look, oftentimes the weight is in kilograms. Unless you're better than me at converting kilograms into pounds, you won't know your weight anyway. I admit I've even been a bit of a rebel in the past and just declined to get on the scale, but I've been informed by a doctor that recording your weight at each visit is required by insurance and Medicaid. It's probably better to be friendly and let them weigh you.

3. Set One Goal (Besides Weight Loss) to Get You Started

You might have bought this book because you want to shed a little (or a lot) of weight. However, for the time being I would like you to take the focus off of a number on the scale. A number is only an external validation of who you are and how you want to feel. So, I'd like to encourage you to go a little upstream from the goal of weight loss. In other words, how would you like to be acting or thinking differently that would ultimately result in you losing weight?

Take a moment to stop and close your eyes while you take a couple of deep breaths. See what answers arise. If you are keeping a journal as you read through the book, write down whatever thoughts or ideas came to your mind. Some answers I often hear are "I'd like to eat slower," "I'd like to stop eating before I'm full," "I'd like to stop eating in front of the computer and while I'm reading," and "I'd like to stop eating the last bites of food on my children's plates."

If nothing occurred to you this time, keep checking in as you continue reading. As you'll discover in the next chapter, the practice of mindfulness can bring new insights and answers to the surface.

WHAT'S IN THE BOOK

Picking up this book means you are choosing to take your own journey to better health. You will actively participate in your own recovery from unhealthy habitual ways of eating and living to the satisfaction of eating with pleasure and embracing the present and all it has to offer. This book will take you through the process, guiding you through these steps:

- discovering the practice of mindfulness and how it directly relates to eating (Chapters 2 and 3)

- understanding how to live with the no-forbidden-food philosophy without going overboard (Chapter 4)

- listening and responding to the thoughts and beliefs that generally lead you to the fridge (Chapter 5)

- learning how to take care of all of your hungers— physical, emotional, mental, and spiritual (Chapter 6)

- learning how to get your body moving in ways that feel delicious (Chapter 7)

- understanding how to make healthy food without it taking too much time or costing too much (Chapter 8)

- experimenting with the tasty world of food while being conscious of where food comes from and the impact your food choices have on you individually and globally (Chapter 9)

- developing a plan for your continued growth and success as a mindful eater (Chapter 10)

You will find exercises in each chapter aimed at helping you learn, practice, and build the skills necessary to accomplish all of these steps. Several of the exercises are available as audio and video downloads on the New Harbinger website (http://www.newharbin ger.com/33278) and my website (http://www.lynnrossy.com).

Of course, there will be challenges with any worthwhile endeavor you undertake. When you notice yourself getting frustrated with the process, remember this is a journey you take one step and one bite at a time. It isn't always easy, but the payoff is well worth the effort. It's about moving from a life lived on automatic pilot to a life lived wide awake.

Be grateful right now for your amazing body and all that it can do. As you start your journey, remember what my mentor says: "As long as you are breathing, there is more right with you than wrong with you" (Kabat-Zinn 2013, xxviii).

CHALLENGES:

- The diet mentality is ingrained in our cultural psyche. It is very clever and sometimes hard to detect.

- It is hard not to give in to the next new diet that promises to work.

- Mindless eating is supported by many environmental, physical, and emotional cues.

- Reconnecting to the wisdom of the body is a journey and doesn't happen overnight.

THE GOOD NEWS:

- The end of the struggle with food and your body starts with mindfulness—a kind and curious attention to the present.

- You inner guidance will lead you to better health and happiness.

- Loving food, in and of itself, is not a problem if you also love the way you feel after you eat it.

- When you savor your food (particularly the cake), you can enjoy it fully without having more than you need.

WHAT YOU CAN DO NOW:

- Get off the diets.

- Get off the scale.

- Set one goal (besides weight loss) to get you started.

CHAPTER 2

Taking Your Life Off Automatic Pilot

Mindfulness is getting a lot of attention these days—and for good reason. Thousands of people hungry for answers to their challenges with food, weight, and stress of every kind are finding mindfulness to be of tremendous help. If you look at the statistics from Google, searches for the term *mindfulness* have grown dramatically in the past couple of years. Mindfulness is popping up like Starbucks coffee shops in every corner around the world.

The increasing interest from the American public, trendsetters, influential leaders, major corporations, and scientists led *Huffington Post* senior writer Carolyn Gregoire to recently suggest that "mindfulness will change the world" and you in the process. More than a trend, the mindfulness movement is a recognition of our need for balance and sanity. Maybe your life hasn't been touched by mindfulness yet, but that is just about to change.

Before I talk about mindfulness, this chapter will discuss its opposite—mindlessness—and the consequences it has on the way you eat and live your life. From there, you will be introduced to mindfulness—what it is, why it's important, how it's practiced, and how you can use it to your benefit starting today.

MINDLESSNESS

Mindlessness is an experience we can all relate to. Have you ever walked into a room and forgotten why you were there? Have you ever been driving somewhere and forgotten where you were going? Have you ever been looking everywhere for the glasses that were resting on top of your head? These are just a few examples of when we operate without our minds being engaged in our moment-to-moment activities. Understanding when and how mindlessness happens and acknowledging the impact it has on your life will be helpful as you learn to move toward a more mindful way of eating and living.

Living on Automatic Pilot

Mindlessness, or mindless behavior, is often described as being on "automatic pilot." It starts as soon as the alarm clock goes off in the morning. You go through your daily routine to get ready for work (have coffee, shower, dress), get the kids ready for school ("Get up and get dressed"), and have breakfast (your daily cereal and banana). You drive to work along the same route (and you even drive there on Saturday when you meant to go somewhere else). You eat everything on your plate, even if you're not hungry (because you were told to do so when you were a child). You probably fall into familiar patterns at work, and at least of few of them (regularly checking social media, surfing the web, and gossiping) are not helping you get your work done.

Mindlessness is reinforced by the frenetic pace and structure of the modern world. Everyone I talk to admits to being too busy and usually quite distracted. We are on information and activity overload, so we try desperately to multitask our way through life. Because our brains aren't designed with the ability to be present to more than one thing at a time, we end up giving our partial attention to everything—sometimes called *continuous partial attention*. Under these circumstances, mindlessness prevails.

The problems that arise from living in a hyperkinetic environment are described by Edward Hallowell, a psychiatrist who has diagnosed and treated thousands of people with attention-deficit/ hyperactivity disorder (ADHD). He coined the term attention deficit trait, or ADT—which, unlike its cousin, ADHD, is caused by brain overload and presents with symptoms including distractibility, inner frenzy, and impatience. At the workplace, ADT shows up as the inability to stay organized, set priorities, and manage time (Hallowell 2005). As our minds fill beyond capacity, the brain gradually loses its ability to attend fully and thoroughly to anything. If you live in a modern culture, you will be affected by an attention deficit and resulting mindlessness.

Eating on Automatic Pilot

Patty, who admitted to always doing something else while she ate, came to understand the consequences of multitasking. She said, "I thought my inability to stay with a diet, eat healthy, or have the body I wanted was due to my lack of self-discipline and no staying power. If you're not aware of what you're doing and your mind is somewhere else, it is next to impossible for you to eat and live the way you'd like to. Now I know my inability to 'stay on track' had to do with a lack of awareness, or mindfulness."

Think about it a moment. Do you ever *just eat*? If you're like most people, eating has become one of those things you do when you're working at the computer, watching TV, reading, or even driving! You eat while you're socializing or sitting in meetings. You eat while you're thinking about what you need to get done, who you're mad at, or what new pair of shoes you want to buy. The concept of *just eating* may be quite foreign to you at this point.

Occupied by the multitude of distractions and demands for your attention, you don't even think about stopping to notice and savor the food in front of you. You generally don't check in to see if you're hungry before you eat. And when you do eat, you don't pay attention to the signals that you're getting full—and end up eating too much. You often don't truly taste the food you eat and have a hard time recalling what you ate at your last meal. If any of these behaviors resemble your life, don't worry, this is not a form of dementia, but a simple lack of attention. Living from the neck up, it's easy to forget about your body throughout the day unless it has some kind of pain that grabs your attention.

And, according to marketing research, when you're not paying attention, you can be easily influenced by small cues around you such as "family and friends, packages and plates, names and numbers, labels and light, colors and candles, shapes and smells, distractions and distances, cupboards and containers" (Buettner 2008, 229). According to Wansink and Sobal (2007), people make nearly twenty times more daily decisions about food than they are aware of (an average of around 250 each day!). Multiple industries (e.g., advertising firms, flavor companies, food product developers, food manufacturers) are working around the clock to grab your attention to eat the food they're selling, and they're banking on the fact that you're not really paying attention.

Author Cheri Huber (2007, 4) writes, "We don't lack self-discipline, we lack presence." And apparently "presence" (or attention) is something that humans have been lacking for a long time. Over five hundred years ago, Leonardo da Vinci described the average person as one who "looks without seeing, listens without hearing, touches without feeling, eats without tasting, moves without awareness of odor or fragrances, and talks without thinking" (Gelb 2010, 27).

This is a perfect description of mindless eating and living. Do you find your head nodding in recognition of how you live way too much of the time? Just pause a moment to consider the consequences of mindlessness and you can quickly comprehend the negative effects, particularly when it comes to eating.

EATING WITHOUT TASTING

When you "eat without tasting," there are a few things that occur. First, you miss out on the wonderful tastes the world of food has to offer. Because of your tendency to live on automatic pilot, you fall into habits with food that limit the variety of what you eat. Unless you consciously browse the wonderful world of food, you can't believe the tastes you're missing out on. Even simple food becomes delicious when you fully bring your attention to it.

Second, when you eat without tasting, you are probably consuming food that isn't enjoyable out of habit. I told you earlier about Karen, who discovered she didn't like anything she ate on a regular basis. So, believe it or not, you may be consuming food you don't like and that your wise body would rather reject. I'm always heartened by the stories people share when they bring a fresh curiosity to how their food tastes. Lately I've been hearing a surprising number of stories about people using their new skill of mindfulness at Dairy Queen. They were all convinced that mindfulness would not change how they experienced their beloved Blizzard. However, when they put the Blizzard to the test of mindful eating, they threw at least half of it away because it "didn't really taste like food" and wasn't nearly as good as they thought it was going to be.

Third, when you eat without tasting, you probably overeat. When you are doing other things and your mind is focused on something else, it's as if your brain doesn't register the fact that you've eaten. Under these conditions, it's hard to hear your body's signals that say "I'm satisfied." You don't stop until the food is all gone, regardless of how much is in front of you and whether you wanted or needed so much.

ARE YOU A MINDLESS EATER?

Do you eat when you're reading, watching TV, or sitting in front of a computer? Do you eat when you're stressed, bored, lonely, angry, happy, or tired? Do you eat just because there's food sitting around? Do you eat when you're not hungry? Do you eat because the clock says it's time for breakfast, lunch, or dinner? Do you eat until you're uncomfortable or stuffed? Do you forget what you had to eat at your last meal? Do you eat for a quick pleasure or comfort fix? If you answered yes to any or all of those questions, congratulations! You can officially join the huge club of mindless eaters.

Why Are We So Mindless?

It isn't your fault! You can blame it on your brain. Yes, according to neuroscientists, we are made this way. As they describe it, the brain operates on two networks—the *default mode* network and the *direct experience* network. Mainly we operate on default. Instead of living in the present, we're usually lost in thought—ruminating about the past, worrying about the future, making our to-do lists, or being lost in a daydream. Again, this is our default and it takes some effort not to fall prey to it most of the time.

To demonstrate this, a recent study from Harvard used an iPhone app to gather 250,000 data points on subjects' thoughts, feelings, and actions as they went about their lives. What the researchers discovered is that people are lost in thought about 50 percent of the time. Further, the more time we spend in our heads, the less happy and more anxious we become (Killingsworth and Gilbert 2010). This tendency to *not* be present has been linked not only to depression and anxiety, but also to ADHD and Alzheimer's disease. The effects of mindlessness go even further, creating a plethora of problems from forgetting what you wanted to get at the grocery store to major relationship breakdowns. And, of course, when you're not paying attention, you are more likely to end up saying things like "I can't believe I ate the whole thing!"

MINDFULNESS TO THE RESCUE

Given the fact that you are distracted, busy, and overworked, it is not surprising that you might be overlooking the best source of wisdom you have available to you (and it's right under your nose)—your own body, mind, and heart in the present moment. Accessing that wisdom is made possible through waking up to the present by developing the skill of mindfulness. Mindfulness gives you an alternative to living life on default and guides you to a more conscious way of eating and living. "You have to be present to win," as it says on the raffle ticket. And, as it turns out, being present is not only the condition for winning the raffle, but the key to everything from healthy eating to greater health and happiness.

Mindfulness helps you be present with a curious, accepting attitude of your thoughts, feelings, and body sensations as well as the experiences around you that occur every moment. The reason mindfulness is the key to changing behavior, finding peace with food, and being happier is that it helps you become unhooked from your mind's constant wandering (default mode network) while at the same time activating parts of the brain involved in monitoring and controlling your thoughts and behaviors (Brewer et al. 2011).

Apply this ability to monitor your behavior to the act of eating. When you take that extra nanosecond for mindful awareness before reaching for the candy, you have time to ask yourself whether candy is what you really want. Does it look good? Are you hungry for a little treat or searching to fix your feelings of frustration and impatience? Do you want it just because it's in your line of sight? Are you reaching for it out of habit? Sometimes you'll still have your candy, but you'll be aware of it, have less of it, and enjoy it more when you do. Ultimately you learn to respond more wisely and skillfully.

When we experience life through all of the sights, sounds, smells, tastes, touches, and thoughts that are happening in each successive moment, the direct experience network of the brain is activated. When you are paying attention to the sensory information available in the present, you tend to be less caught up in what happened in the past or in your habits, expectations, or assumptions.

This makes you more responsive to the world around you as it's happening *now*.

Here's Holly's story. She was having difficulty managing her diabetes because of her inability to make the right food choices and balance her food intake. After two weeks of practicing mindfulness, she wrote, "I have been doing the mindfulness exercises only out of obligation over the course of two weeks. I did not actually think of them as doing me any good until one day as I was 'checking in with myself' [which is part of mindfulness practice] and began to realize that I have been allowing outside forces to control me and my eating lifestyle rather than listening to what my 'self' actually needs. I operate in crisis mode because it is the only thing I have ever known when it comes to taking care of myself. I realized that I do have time to take care of myself, to listen to what I need now, to prepare healthy meals and exercise, to get the sleep I need and to ponder upon what I feel. This was a *huge* revelation."

Mindfulness is indeed a "huge revelation" to everybody who starts to practice it, and it can quickly make significant differences in how you lead your life. A wise teacher of mine said, "I practice mindfulness so I don't have an accidental life." Lord knows I wish I would have heard this advice when I was younger! I might have made some different choices. But, like me, most of us were never taught how to listen to our internal wisdom about what, when, why, and how much to eat. Even more startling, most of us weren't taught to listen to our internal wisdom for making decisions in other important areas of our lives either—or even just to pause for a moment to take a breath as we career from one activity to another.

Like Holly, you will discover that, living in the present moment with mindfulness, you can learn to make the choices, think the thoughts, and take the actions that honor you and the life you were meant to live.

Mindfulness Defined

The often-cited definition of mindfulness by Jon Kabat-Zinn (1994, 4), who pioneered the field of mindfulness-based programs decades ago, is "paying attention in a particular way: on purpose, in the present moment, and nonjudgmentally." This moment-to-moment process has been theorized by Shapiro and colleagues (2006) to have three fundamental building blocks, or core components, that occur simultaneously:

1. "On purpose," or *intention*

2. "Paying attention," or *attention*

3. "In a particular way," or *attitude*

Let's break those pieces down one at a time.

COMPONENT #1: INTENTION

We shouldn't underestimate the power of intention for helping us show up and create the life we want. Since we tend to be awfully distracted most of the time, setting an intention (on purpose) to be present is the first important step. Otherwise, unless something is extraordinarily engaging, living in the here and now is unlikely to happen. An intention and personal vision helps to remind you why you are practicing mindfulness and sets the stage for what is possible. Intentions might include being able to better regulate your food intake, enjoy your food more, or have a healthier body. Research indicates that people just starting to practice mindfulness often do so with the intention of self-regulation. Over time their intention tends to develop to include a broader self-exploration (Shapiro 1992). The goal you set in the previous chapter is an example of an intention and can help you in your efforts to keep coming back to the present moment.

COMPONENT #2: ATTENTION

Once you've connected with your intentions, you still have quite a bit of work to do. As I mentioned earlier, mind wandering is our default and being in the present is something we have to develop. The good news is that our brains can be trained to get better at this. Your job is to keep bringing your attention back to what's happening right now—what you're hearing, seeing, feeling, touching, smelling, and thinking. When your mind wanders from what's happening right now, you bring it back. Your mind will wander a thousand times, and your job is to bring your attention back a thousand times. It's okay; wandering is what the mind does well and it's pretty practiced at doing it.

Don't get discouraged or judge yourself for having a mind that wanders. There is no way to do this wrong. The most important part of the practice is to just notice when you're not present and bring your attention back to what's happening in the present, over and over. The repetition of renewed attention to the present (similar to repetitions with weights to build up your arms) actually builds the brain's capacity to stay in the present more often. It's like going to the gym for your brain. I call it building your "mental musculature."

Think about how this applies to eating. Purposely bringing your attention back to eating after you've been distracted can help you be aware of how the food tastes, whether you enjoy it, and when you're satisfied. Further, it can help you be aware of the underlying thoughts and feelings that drive you to eat when you're not really hungry for food. Let's face it, we will probably all continue to eat while we're doing something else at least some of the time. But, we can bring ourselves back to the eating experience over and over again to keep us in touch with the joy of eating and satisfying our hunger.

COMPONENT #3: ATTITUDE

The third component of mindfulness instructs you in the attitudes to cultivate in relation to all of your experiences and senses in the present moment. Paying attention *nonjudgmentally* means observing everything that arises in the moment—the things you like and the things you don't like—with impartial curiosity, kindness, and acceptance. While paying attention with intention is pretty revealing and healing, paying attention without judgment can radically alter your life. This aspect of mindfulness adds a whole new level of complexity to the practice and will be something to undertake with patience.

When I first started on the path of mindfulness, I attended a weekend meditation retreat where I had ample opportunity to listen to how I was relating to the present and everything in it. I was horrified at how much criticism and judgment my mind engaged in *constantly*. In fact, it was quite painful to discover what my mind was saying a lot of the time. I came to the conclusion that either a very nasty monster had taken over my mind or I had been like this all my life and I just hadn't noticed before. Neither proposition was very comforting. About a month later, with tears in my eyes, I had the opportunity to ask some wise mindfulness teachers what I should do. They told me not to worry. "It's not a problem," they said. "Everyone's mind is like that. Just allow it to be as it is." I wasn't very happy about the response at the time, but I eventually learned to bring an attitude of curiosity and kindness—even to my critical mind.

Here are some important things to remember as you begin to encounter your mind with mindfulness. First, everyone has a critical mind. Don't be surprised when you encounter yours. When judgments arise, you simply notice them. Second, you don't have to believe the judgments that arise in your mind. Believe it or not, your thoughts are usually not accurate. Third, when you stop struggling with your mind, you feel a whole lot better.

At first, this act of impartial observation can be quite difficult to practice since we are often feeling some resistance to the way things are in the present moment. The practice of mindfulness asks you to move from this opposition into a relationship with the present that allows it to be just as it is. For instance, if you're experiencing an uncomfortable feeling such as anxiety or worry, you simply bring an open, accepting attention to it. You don't need to change it. You can learn to be with it as you gain a better understanding of what it is and how and why it comes and goes. This is a radical shift for most people. In my experience, it took a good year before I really understood that it was okay to have judgments and there was a way of being with them that neutralized their sting.

When you check in with your relationship to the present, what do you notice? If you are experiencing something pleasant and appetizing, you might notice a greedy, grasping attitude (*I want more of it*). If you are experiencing something unpleasant, your attitude could be one of resisting, rejecting, or judging (*I don't want it*). If the present is neither pleasant nor unpleasant, you might zone out, disconnect, or fall asleep (*I'm bored*). Alternatively, if you bring an affectionate attention to the present moment, you can meet all of these states of mind with calm curiosity. Being aware of our relationship to the present is such an important part of the practice of mindfulness (and a key to happiness) that I will be emphasizing it often and giving you practices to strengthen it.

In sum, mindfulness is "affectionate attention" and teaches us to befriend the moment and ourselves exactly as we are. That's why I like to define mindfulness as "being present with all of one's senses with curiosity and kindness."

Practicing Mindfulness

Although it's estimated that we only live in the present a small percentage of the time, the good news is that we can strengthen our ability to be here more often. There are specific ways of learning the skill of mindfulness and how to put it to use in your life. A purely intellectual understanding of mindfulness will never reap the benefits of first-hand experience.

Just as with anything you want to get good at, you have to practice it. If you want to cook well, you need to experiment and practice with different kinds of foods and spices. If you want to run a marathon, you have to run regularly. If you want to learn how to play the piano well, you have to practice your scales and musical pieces. If you want to be in the present more often, there are formal and informal ways of improving this as well.

To highlight the importance of practice, I often tell the story of Pablo Casals, one of the greatest cellists of all time. When asked at age ninety-three why he continued to practice the cello three hours a day, he responded, "I'm beginning to notice some improvement." You will be able to see improvement in your ability to be mindful from the very beginning—even after two attempts. But just think of what you might discover if you practice every day until you're ninety-three!

First of all, engaging in formal mindfulness practice sets the stage for bringing mindfulness into every aspect of your life. The formal practices of mindfulness include sitting meditation with awareness of the breath, the body scan (scanning your body sensations from head to toe), loving-kindness (offering kind wishes to yourself and others), and mindful yoga. These practices help build up your mental musculature so that you can be present more often. As I said before, it's sort of like going to the gym for your mind, except unlike the gym, there are no special clothes, shoes, or gym memberships to buy. You just need to give yourself the gift of a little time each day to see positive results. To get you started, there are instructions in this chapter for a short mindfulness practice called A Taste of Mindfulness. Then, each chapter in the book will give you a new formal practice to add to your repertoire.

Second, you take the "attention muscle" that you build in formal practice and put it to use as you go about your day. You can practice being mindful from the moment you wake up until the moment you go to sleep at night (although I'm not sure anyone has ever accomplished that feat!). Instead of shifting into automatic pilot during routine activities like showering, walking, driving, making your bed, sweeping the floor, cooking, or eating, you can bring a curious, kind attention to what it actually feels like to be alive in these moments. This is often called informal mindfulness practice and doesn't take any extra time out of your day. It just requires that you shift your attention from being lost in thought to fully engaging in these activities. In a sense, you can turn your whole life into a meditation.

I taught the short mindfulness exercise described below to a group of 350 women at a health conference. Afterward, I asked everyone to share something about what they noticed. One woman who had never practiced mindfulness before opened her eyes and exclaimed, "All of the colors in the room look brighter!" I assure you no one had repainted the room in the three minutes she had her eyes closed, but she woke up to her surroundings and the sensation of color. Even the otherwise mundane parts of your life can become extraordinary.

Exercise: A Taste of Mindfulness

Are you ready for what you might discover? Let's get started with a short practice you can do throughout your day. It's one of the most powerful exercises you'll learn, and it's the quickest and easiest to do. Please read the instructions below and take your time to practice it. You can also download and listen to an audio recording of A Taste of Mindfulness on the New Harbinger website, http://www.newhar binger.com/33278 (or at http://www.lynnrossy.com).

Start by sitting in a comfortable position, with an erect yet relaxed posture. Close your eyes or have a soft gaze down at the floor. Start by taking a couple of deep breaths—let your belly be soft and full as you breathe in, and expel all of the air as you breath out. Gradually let the breath become natural and effortless. Feel the movement of the belly, the ribcage, and the chest in response to the air coming into and out of the body.

Now, scan your body from head to toe—notice the current state of your body. Are there places of tension? Places that feel relaxed? What parts of your body feel warm or cool? Is the body energized or fatigued? Just notice what is present. Take your time.

Pay particular attention to the sensations at the area of the stomach. Are there sensations of hunger? Of satiety? How hungry or full are you? Are you thirsty? You might notice thoughts of judgment about your stomach. Just let those come and go.

Next, notice what feelings are present. You might be feeling curious, angry, happy, frustrated, confused, or content. No matter what feelings are present, acknowledge them with curiosity and kindness.

Notice what thoughts are passing through your mind. Let thoughts arise, exist, and pass away without getting caught up in the story of the thoughts as best you can.

You might notice how the feelings and thoughts are connected. If you are feeling restless, you might have thoughts about needing to get something done, or if you're feeling angry, you might be having thoughts about someone who upsets you. Just notice what's present without judging.

When you know what your body feels like, what feelings are present, and what thoughts are going through your head, you've dropped out of automatic pilot.

For a couple more moments, sit and breathe and experience what it means to be alive in this moment. When your mind gets lost in a story, bring your attention back to the passing sensations that are available in the present moment—body, breath, sounds. It doesn't matter how many times the mind wanders. The important thing is to notice, without judgment, and bring your attention back. Each time the mind wanders and you notice it is a moment of waking up to the present.

Notice that some things you experience feel pleasant and some not so pleasant. No matter what you're experiencing, allowing each moment to be exactly as it is and allowing yourself to be exactly as you are. Sitting, breathing, and simply being. And, when you're ready, opening your eyes.

What did you notice?

After you open your eyes and end the exercise, take a moment to reflect on what you noticed. If you have a notebook or journal, write these down. What body sensations did you notice? What feelings did you notice? What thoughts did you notice? What other experiences were you aware of?

_____

Be curious, like a scientist would be when examining something for the first time. Remember, every time you examine your inner experience will be a little different. No moment is the same as the next. And, there is no right way to feel or be. All experiences, inside and outside of you, are welcomed and allowed. In this way, mindfulness helps you to befriend all things.

Common experiences that people report when engaging in this exercise include restlessness, sleepiness, worry, doubt, aversion, and pleasure. You might have felt one or all of these states in one sitting. You might have become aware of tension or pain in your shoulders, back, or neck that you weren't aware of until you closed your eyes and tuned in to the body. I actually have people accuse me of causing them pain by teaching them meditation! But, believe it or not, the pain was always there—the exercise didn't cause it—and not noticing it before is a validation of how out of touch we are with our bodies much of the time. Often, upon noticing the tension or pain, you might experience a slight to significant release and relaxing of your muscles. You might have noticed your breath getting deeper just by bringing your attention to it.

It would not be surprising if you noticed a *lot* of thinking going on—a recitation of the to-do list, anxieties and worries, daydreams, or just random thoughts about nothing all that important. On the other hand, you might have had an interesting insight about an issue you haven't resolved.

If you think you can't do this "mindfulness thing" because your mind wanders, don't worry. This is not true! Everybody's mind wanders. That's why it's often referred to as the "monkey mind." Our thoughts are jumping around like monkeys flying through the trees from limb to limb. Instead of being distracted by all of these thoughts, mindfulness teaches us to be aware of what our mind is thinking but not lost in the stories it concocts all the time.

This ability to be aware of the thinking process is called *meta-awareness*. You simply know you're thinking and you're aware of the contents of your thoughts without adding judgment, decision, or commentary. In this way, you can begin to become familiar with your favorite patterns of thinking such as planning, worrying, complaining, and criticizing. Avoiding having your attention captured by these common types of automatic thoughts can require continuous monitoring because the mind is almost constantly chattering away.

Remember, there is also no "right" way to feel when you practice mindfulness. You can feel and notice all kinds of things. The important thing is to simply acknowledge how things are for you in this moment. Through this simple act of tuning in to yourself like you would tune in to a radio station, you can hear what kind of music is playing inside and take the pulse of your human experience. When you turn on the radio, sometimes you'll like what the station is playing and sometimes you won't. While you can change the radio station if you don't like the music, you can't always change the way you're feeling. However, just by naming and acknowledging what's happening, particularly when it's unpleasant, you begin to cultivate a partnership with yourself that is kind and healing.

Since I know that starting and engaging in mindfulness practice can be a real challenge, particularly when you are on your own and learning it from a book, I need to inquire: did you actually *do* the Taste of Mindfulness exercise, or did you just read it and perhaps *imagine* what it would be like to do it? If you didn't actually do it, please go back and do it now. Mindfulness is the key—the foundation—to your success, and it's something that can only be learned experientially, not intellectually. Give yourself the gift of actually trying it. I will wait for you while you go back and do it.

Making Time for Practice

A Taste of Mindfulness is an essential tool for getting back in touch with yourself. Once you've checked in, you have a better idea of how to navigate your life. Just a little mindfulness is sometimes all you need to tap into the body's wisdom about when and what to eat, when to move and when to stretch, when to rest, when to play, when to work, and how to respond to a myriad of other needs or desires.

You can do this exercise anywhere and anytime: before you eat, when you're walking down the street, when you're in a meeting, when you're feeling stressed or upset, when you're in between activities or projects, when you're cooking dinner, or even when you're making love. I've had students tell me they even do it while they're driving. If you do that though, please remember to keep your eyes open!

Now that you've done A Taste of Mindfulness (and I truly hope you did), think for a moment about when would be a good time for you to practice. I suggest picking three times over the course of the day so that you can sprinkle your day with mindfulness. Write down the times in your journal, if you are keeping one, or you can write down your times on a sticky note and post it in a prominent place. There is a great power in setting an intention, and writing it down can help you stay on track. You can even make a commitment out loud to a trusted friend or family member.

Read the Warning Label

Once you begin to practice mindfulness and become more awake for your life, you will never be able to live as unconsciously as you did in the past. In other words, there's no turning back. You will begin to sense the difference between living on automatic pilot and living in the present. You will be more acutely aware of when you are thinking and behaving in ways that are not consistent with the person you want to be. You will also be more available to the wonderful pleasures of being alive—including the joy of eating.

Cathy, a busy mother of three and a lifelong dieter, put it this way: "I can honestly say that learning mindfulness has been a life-changing experience. I never realized how stuck I was until now. I really feel as if many things are illuminated just by quietly turning my attention to them. It is so amazing how mindfulness has become infused into all aspects of my life."

The key to the relationship you want with your food, your body, and your life lies in your commitment to be present more often. Waking up to each moment is the only way you can savor and appreciate the food you eat, honor and support the body you have, and create the life you want. Don't miss out!

CHALLENGES:

- Remembering to be present isn't easy when you are caught in the *default mode* network of the brain.

- About half of the time you are lost in thought—worrying about the future, ruminating about the past, making your to-do lists, or being lost in a daydream.

- When you're lost in thought, you tend to be more depressed and anxious.

- The more distracted you are, the more you will eat mindlessly.

- When you "eat without tasting," you enjoy your food less, eat food that you don't even like, and overeat.

THE GOOD NEWS:

- Mindfulness is the key to changing behavior, finding peace with food, and being happier.

- You can activate the *direct experience* network of the brain by being present to the world around you as it's happening in the moment and being a better monitor of your body, feelings, thoughts, and behavior.

- Mindfulness practice helps you to set skillful intentions, be present, and cultivate attitudes of nonjudgment, kindness, curiosity, and acceptance.

- You can strengthen your ability to be mindfully present in any moment through practice—both formal and informal.

WHAT YOU CAN DO NOW:

- A Taste of Mindfulness: Do this exercise three times a day at the times you designated. You can also do it anytime you need to take a purposeful pause to check in with yourself.

CHAPTER 3

The BASICS of Mindful Eating

By bringing to light the major difficulties and challenges you have with eating, the instructions in this chapter will transform your future experiences with food and your body. There is no great mystery or secret to unveil, just the simple task of bringing your attention to what's happening in the present. When you're on autopilot—not paying attention to what you're doing or being fully present in your body—you're not aware of the sensations of hunger or fullness, not aware of what you're eating, and not tasting or enjoying your food. Conditioned thoughts and unconscious decisions and choices create a war between you and your food and body, but they are not the enemy. When the present is experienced directly and your thoughts and habits are recognized, new choices become available that honor your taste buds and your health. You can befriend and delight in the experience of tasting, eating, and living. Here are the "basics" that can change what, when, why, and how you eat.

BASICS OF MINDFUL EATING

Now that you know a little bit about mindfulness, we are going to take that knowledge and apply it to eating. BASICS is an acronym for a complete set of guidelines that walk you through the eating process from beginning to end. They will teach you how to be present with food and your body before you eat, while you're eating, and as you determine when to stop eating. These are not rules, and it would be foolhardy to think you could follow them perfectly all of the time. However, practicing the BASICS will change the way you eat forever and for the better—training you how to eat for pleasure and health. They will be your touchstone for the rest of your eating life.

BASICS stands for:

B—Breathe and belly check for hunger and satiety before you eat

A—Assess your food

S—Slow down

I—Investigate your hunger throughout the meal, particularly halfway through

C—Chew your food thoroughly

S—Savor your food

Let's talk about them one at a time.

B—Breathe and belly check for hunger and satiety before you eat

BASIC INSTRUCTIONS: First, take a few deep breaths and relax the body. As you're doing this, check in with your belly. Are there sensations of physical hunger? How hungry are you? What are you hungry for? Is there a particular type of food you'd like to have? You might want food. You might be thirsty. You might be hungry for something entirely different from food (e.g., walking, stretching, more deep breaths, relief from stress). Listen to what your body is telling you. General rule: eat when you're hungry; don't eat when you're not hungry.

Most of us are barely breathing, which is why the first instruction is so important. Notice how you're breathing right now. You will probably discover that you're holding some tension in your belly. Relax and let it go. Take a few deep breaths. Let your belly be soft and allow the breath to be deep and full. Notice how different it is to breathe this way. To change the habit of shallow breathing, it can be helpful to take a few deep breaths throughout the day. Breathing deeply is essential for your journey back to your body and will improve your understanding and recognition of hunger and satiety cues. I find it a little humorous that I got a Ph.D. to go around teaching people to breathe, but it truly is a prescription for better health and well-being. And the best news is that it's free and available at every moment.

Besides the obvious fact that you need to breathe in order to live, when your breath is shallow it may be a symptom of stress. The more shallow your breathing is, the more stressed and anxious you will feel. Symptoms of stress include muscle tension, rapid heartbeat, clenched jaw, shakiness, upset stomach, cold or sweaty hands and feet, dry mouth, and difficulty swallowing. These symptoms are indications that you have been triggered with the fight-or-flight response. And if you think you are not at risk, it's estimated that the average American gets triggered with a brief stress response an average of fifty times a day (Domar and Dreher 1996)—often starting when the alarm clock goes off in the morning!

When you're stressed, your body's resources are being utilized to escape a real or imagined threat. When triggered, the fight-or-flight mechanisms in the body can override your brain's capacity to make good decisions. As a result, you easily fall into habitual behavior that often includes reaching for food. One of the reasons you turn to food is because stress induces secretion of glucocorticoids, which increases the desire for food, and insulin, which promotes food intake. Eating actually reduces the stress response and reinforces your tendency to eat when stressed (Dallman 2010). Due to these mechanisms, stress and obesity are, not surprisingly, linked together.

In addition, when you eat when you're stressed, your body stores more food as fat. And, my guess is, storing extra fat is not the outcome you are hoping for. Interestingly enough, the body is actually preparing you to be without food for a while, maybe while you're hiding in a cave as you take cover from your enemies. This bodily process is part of our survival mechanism and made sense when we had to hide from lions, tiger, and bears, but now it just makes us fat!

Ever find yourself reaching for food when you get angry, frustrated, irritated, afraid, or stressed? Your body is really asking for relief from tension, and food has probably provided some temporary relief in the past. However, when food is sought out as the answer to an emotional state, you end up eating junk you don't need and you're still left with your original problem.

Alternatively, when you breathe deeply and you're in a relaxed state, you're able to metabolize your food more efficiently. You breathe in more oxygen and you burn food more fully. When you take a few deep breaths, the parasympathetic nervous system kicks in, reversing the signs of stress in the body and alleviating the desire to reach for food. Try a little deep breathing to bring your body's natural resources to the rescue. Over time you will begin to recognize the difference between the symptoms of stress and the physical symptoms of hunger.

When you check in with your belly, see if you notice physical symptoms such as mild gurgling or grumbling in the stomach, representing biological hunger and the body's actual need for nutrients. If you ignore the first signs of hunger, the body continues to speak to you through other symptoms such as irritability, difficulty concentrating, light-headedness, stomach pain, headaches, lack of energy, and faintness.

As you can see, some symptoms of stress could easily be confused with hunger symptoms. However, symptoms of stress are caused by feelings and thoughts, and symptoms of hunger are caused by not having been fed for a while. Eventually you can begin to sense the difference. Every uncomfortable feeling that you have in your body is not hunger nor should be fixed with food. So instead of reaching for a bag of chips or a chocolate bar, take a breath and check in to see what your body is telling you. Stay tuned, because we will talk much more about stress and emotional eating in a later chapter.

Because you are accustomed to eating for many reasons besides hunger, the idea of checking in with your belly to see if you're hungry before you eat might be a somewhat foreign idea for you. You may be out of touch with the signs of hunger or how to interpret the signals from your belly. As a result, you might be skeptical about anything your belly tells you. Truth be told, you might be ignoring your belly for all kinds of reasons. I often hear statements like "Check in with my belly?!" "I don't like my belly!" "How can I trust a belly that just tells me to eat all of the time?"

This is when mindfulness comes to the rescue. Take a few more deep breaths and bring the focus to your belly with nonjudgmental curiosity and kindness. This caring attention is an essential attitude to cultivate as you learn to improve your relationship with your body. It may take some time, but your belly *can* become your buddy. Start by breathing and relaxing. Bring an interested, caring attention to the present moment and tune in to the sensations in the belly. Ask yourself, "Am I hungry?"

As you learn to explore your hunger, here is a scale you can use to help you determine how hungry or full you are. Used regularly, it can teach you the language of hunger.

Hunger and Satisfaction Scale

1. Starved! I don't care what or how much I eat!

2. Very hungry! I feel unfocused and irritable.

3. Hungry—I feel a physical sense of hunger.

4. Slightly hungry

5. Not hungry, but not yet satisfied

6.   Satisfied with the meal

7.   Starting to get a feeling of fullness

8.   A little too full, feeling uncomfortable

9.   Way too full! I couldn't eat another bite.

10. Stuffed! I feel sick!

Each time before you eat, ask yourself: "Am I hungry? What's my hunger level?" The first step to reclaiming the world of normal eating is to honor your biological hunger. Your body needs to *consistently* know that it will have access to food. If you are starved (number 1), you definitely have waited too long to eat and might eat everything in the house or the grocery store! Sometimes people call this being "hangry!" When you are very hungry (number 2), you feel irritable and unfocused, and your body and brain are exhibiting signs of not having food for too long. The best time to eat is when you have signs of physical hunger in the form of hunger pangs and stomach growling (number 3).

If you wait until you feel physical hunger before you eat, you will still feel slightly hungry (number 4) at the beginning of your meal or snack. As you continue to eat, the hunger will dissipate but you won't feel satisfied (number 5). The place where you do feel satisfied (number 6) is an ideal place to stop eating. At this point your biological hunger needs have been met.

By the time you start feeling a sensation of fullness (number 7), if you eat any more it will probably be too much. When you start to feel uncomfortable (number 8), way too full (number 9), and stuffed (number 10), you can be sure that you are eating way past the point of physical need.

Not being hungry before you eat and being too full when you finish eating are signs that you are engaging in mindless, unconscious eating or eating to fulfill emotional needs. Use this scale to help you better understand and regulate your behavior with food. Checking in with your belly will give you important information about hunger and fullness. As you begin to eat more mindfully, you will notice that eating past the point of biological need is not that pleasant or desirable. The more you acknowledge the discomfort you feel in the body when you eat too much, the more likely you will choose not to feel this way.

Don't be discouraged if you haven't yet discovered how to eat based on your body's messages. Listening, understanding, and honoring your hunger and satiety cues are some of the more challenging aspects of mindful eating, particularly if you haven't been paying attention to your body for a long time. This is perfectly normal at the beginning of your path of mindful eating. For instance, you might have difficulty noticing the signs of hunger, never feel hungry, or feel hungry all of the time. Let's look at a these issues in more detail.

Do you have difficulty feeling hunger or never feel hungry? There are a number of reasons this happens. And, when you don't recognize hunger, you might also be neglecting the body's other needs (e.g., sleep, movement, water).

- Drinking a lot of diet soda, coffee, and tea can silence hunger. These calorie-free beverages provide a temporary sense of fullness in the stomach and numb the hunger signs.

- A long history of dieting can dampen the hunger cues. Dieters who deny their hunger for a long period of time can subsequently learn to tune out the signals of their growling bellies until the signals finally become hard to recognize.

- Eating according to the time on the clock (e.g., breakfast at 7:00 a.m., lunch at noon, and dinner at 7:00 p.m.) can increase your reliance on an external structure instead of your internal signals and dampen your ability to hear and feel your hunger. Even if you have to eat at a particular time, check in to gauge your hunger level and eat an amount that satisfies the level of need.

- Living a busy, nonstop life can result in a habit of ignoring or suppressing hunger as you focus on being engaged in activity all of the time.

- Spending a lot of time in your head and not in your body can also shut off the body's messages. When you are lost in thought, it is difficult to be aware of the voice for hunger.

Do you feel hungry all of the time? Explore the following explanations to see which ones might be contributing to your growling belly.

- Eating food with little staying power will make you feel hungry sooner than later. Most notably, simple carbohydrates (e.g., refined breads, pastas, and sugary foods) are absorbed quickly into the blood, causing a quick increase in blood sugar and a surge of insulin. Insulin prompts cells to absorb blood sugar for energy or storage, and levels in the bloodstream begin to fall. Your body will think it has run out of fuel and you will feel hungry again as you begin to crave more carbohydrates.

- Not drinking enough water can be a culprit. The lack of hydration can mimic signs of hunger because hunger and thirst signals are controlled in the same part of your brain. Try drinking about sixty-four ounces of water a day to stay hydrated.

- Thinking about food a lot can set off cravings. The thought about food and the desire that arises from that thought are not the same as hunger.

Certain psychological, physical, and environmental conditions can make it difficult to accurately assess your biological hunger—making you feel more or less hungry. If you are depressed or anxious or stressed, you might feel overly hungry or not hungry at all. Some medications can mask the signs of hunger (e.g., medications that cause nausea, ADHD drugs, some diabetes medicines) or increase the feelings of hunger (e.g., some antidepressants and diabetes medicines). Lastly, just the smell of delicious food can get those salivary glands working overtime and induce the urge to eat even when you're not really hungry.

Although my general recommendation is to eat when you're hungry and not eat when you're not hungry, there are a few important exceptions. Consider the following suggestions for becoming a better friend to your body.

Having physical energy is dependent on fuel from what you eat. It is the foundation for health in every area of your life. In order to keep your body running smoothly, it is often recommended that you eat something every four or five hours. Use this as a guide when you are first learning to listen to your body's cues. You don't have to eat a lot. A few nuts, a piece of fruit, or a slice of cheese might be just what your body needs to stay happy until the next meal. Stay tuned for the slight signs of hunger because at first you might miss them.

Some people tell me they never eat breakfast, insisting that eating breakfast makes them hungrier during the rest of the day. However, skipping breakfast in an effort to lose weight doesn't work. Research indicates that you tend to eat more food, not less, at your next meal or you succumb to eating fatty, sugary snacks. In addition, eating breakfast has been associated with better concentration, increased alertness and energy, and a decrease in stomachaches and headaches (Wahlstrom and Begalle 1999). Eating smaller, more frequent meals and eating earlier in the day has actually been correlated with eating less over the course of the day and lower body mass index (de Castro 2004; Song et al. 2005). Skipping any meal, but especially breakfast, can actually make weight control more difficult.

Hungry or not, eat your breakfast—even if it's a piece of fruit, some yogurt or oatmeal, a handful of trail mix, or an energy bar. Breakfast is the most important meal of the day and is a way of recalibrating the body by jumpstarting your metabolism after not eating for the period of time you were asleep. By the end of ten weeks, all of my breakfast skeptics have transformed into breakfast believers and say that it makes them feel better and eat less.

When you know you won't be able to eat for many hours and will feel starved before you have access to food again, you would be well advised to eat a little something even if you aren't hungry. Tribole and Resch (1995) call this "practical hunger." For example, imagine you are going to a movie that starts at 7:00 p.m., and an hour earlier you aren't hungry. Eating a light meal or snack beforehand is a sensible solution and will keep you from feeling starved later.

Breathing deeply and checking in with your belly will change not only how you eat, but also how you relate to yourself and your life. You will begin to discover hunger at more and more subtle levels as you work with this simple but profound practice. Be patient and kind with yourself as you learn how to listen and reestablish your connection to the body. After you determine *if* you are hungry, you will want to inquire *what* you're hungry for. Understanding what the body wants and needs might be immediately evident, or you might need to go on a deeper investigation. The next step in the BASICS will help.

A—Assess your food

BASIC INSTRUCTIONS: What does it look like? Notice the colors of the food. Does it look appealing? What does it smell like? Where does it come from? Is it a food you can recognize (e.g., natural and unprocessed), or is it so highly processed you don't know what it is? Is this the food you really want? You don't have to take a lot of time with this. A brief pause to assess your food can give you lots of information about it. As you take your first bite and continue to eat, reassess your food to see whether your first impressions were correct and whether you really want to keep eating.

After breathing and checking in with your belly to see if you're even hungry, the next step is to assess what you're planning on eating. Do you assess your food before you eat or do you throw it into your mouth without pausing to reflect on what it is? Mindless eating happens very quickly, and before you know it you are eating something just because it's there. Now is a good time to take another look at what you're eating—as if for the first time.

When you assess your food, your senses of sight and smell will help you ascertain a lot about the food you're about to eat. Even before you taste it, you might feel your mouth beginning to water. You can actually get a sense of how healthy the food is by tuning in to the way it looks, smells, and feels in your hand. See if you can sense your body wanting it or not. Imagine this for a moment: what would it feel like to hold an apple or grape in your hand? What would it feel like to hold a cupcake or a bag of French fries? What impressions do different types of food leave you with? Of course when you do this for real, you will be able to feel the texture, smell the odors, and sense the reactions in the body.

If you are used to eating highly processed food, it will be more difficult to use your senses to clearly guide you. First, food housed in hermetically sealed packages is hard to smell, hard to touch, and hard to sense. Second, primitive neurochemical reward centers in the brain are triggered by food (even memories of food) laced with sugar, far, and salt and mimic responses found in people addicted to alcohol, drugs, and cigarettes. As you practice assessing your food before you eat, notice whether you can sense the difference between signs that your body desires a particular food for its health or taste and signs that you have developed a biological craving for it. I like to call the first "body hunger" and the other "brain hunger." For example, you might feel your body saying yes to a fresh apple or grapes because the body desires the nutrients found in them, but you might also hear a yes to a doughnut or a bag of French fries because you have developed a craving for them due to their high sugar and fat content.

Assessing your food does not include an evaluation of calories, carbohydrates, fats, salts, or recommended daily allowances. As you are learning to become a mindful eater, a focus on these aspects of your food distracts you from learning about your food through direct experience. Author, journalist, and food activist Michael Pollan (2004) writes, "we've learned to choose our food by the numbers... relying more heavily on our reading and computational skills than upon our senses." People who "eat by numbers" seem constantly concerned with the products they eat and often guide their eating by the latest fad, diet claim, or medical guru. Although the important scientific recommendations available to us should not be discounted, many people have begun to rely solely on this information and block out their own well of wisdom inside their bodies.

Which sounds more appealing to you?

A ripe, red, fresh tomato

OR

33 calories (3 from fat), 9 milligrams of sodium, 7 grams of carbohydrates (2 grams of dietary fiber and 5 grams of sugar), 2 grams of protein, 30% Vitamin A, 39% Vitamin C, 2% Calcium, 3% Iron

My guess is that most of you would prefer eating a ripe, red, fresh tomato (preferably warmed by the sun and straight off the vine). Assessing your food puts you in touch with the direct experience of the food itself, not a scientific calculation.

As she worked on learning to assess her food, Holly discovered that "healthier and more natural foods are actually more appealing to my senses than processed convenience foods." When she stopped to listen to her body, she noticed that it did not respond very well to nights of eating pizza rolls and drinking the soda she loves. However, the night she made broiled chicken with green beans, a salad, and watermelon, her body responded quite differently. "As I scanned this plate of food, I was amazed to find that all of my senses were thoroughly engaged. It was beautifully colorful, and the watermelon smelled delicious and my mouth watered. The salad was crunchy and colorful and excited my taste and sight. The chicken filled my stomach with warmth and sustenance. The green beans were sweet and reminded me of the home-cooked meals of my childhood."

You will become more sensitive to the body's desire for or rejection of food by assessing it before and while you eat. After seeing and smelling your food, your mindful attention to the taste of food and its effect on your body will begin to direct you to keep eating or not. As you learn to assess your food, don't be surprised if you find yourself making different food choices than in the past.

S—Slow down

BASIC INSTRUCTIONS: Slowing down while you are eating helps you be aware of when you're getting full and when the body's physical hunger is satisfied. Slowing down can help you enjoy your food more fully. Simple methods to help you slow down include putting down your fork or spoon between bites, pausing and taking a breath between bites, and chewing your food completely. If you are eating with others, try talking and listening without having your eating utensil constantly in hand and notice how it changes the pace of the meal.

There are many benefits to slowing down while you eat. In a 2008 study published in the *Journal of the American Dietetic Association*, thirty healthy women were studied on two separate occasions in which they ate at two different rates of speed. When they consumed their meals slowly, they ate significantly fewer calories and drank significantly more water than when they ate at a faster rate. Additionally, they were less likely to feel satiated when they ate quickly (Andrade, Greene, and Melanson 2008).

Slowing down and bringing your attention to the food you're eating will help you get the very most out of your eating experience. Of course, one of the best payoffs for slowing down is how it increases your ability to taste and savor your food. We'll talk more about "Savor" at the end of the BASICS, but you can start by learning to take your time when you eat.

For many of us, slowing down will not be an easy practice to learn. How many times have you scarfed down an entire meal and didn't even know what you consumed or how it tasted? Rena said she remembered the night in college when she and her roommate walked down five flights of stairs to the cafeteria, ate dinner, and walked back to their room in less than five minutes. You might not have ever eaten quite that fast, but you get the point.

Eating meals slowly becomes particularly challenging when we're under time constraints, when we eat with other people, and when we find ourselves around environmental influences such as loaded buffet tables and break rooms at work filled with goodies. If you are caring for the never-ending needs of children, it can seem impossible to take time for yourself to eat slowly. Eating often occurs while you're running from the kitchen to the table or from the house to the soccer field.

When you begin to pay attention to your rate of eating, you might also begin to notice how fast other people eat—particularly someone you live with. This can be quite an eye-opener. Watch as people attack and devour their food in moments. As you begin the process of slowing down, fast feels really out of sync. Perhaps you could introduce your fellow diners to the idea of slowing down.

If you're a fast eater, you might be like me—doing a lot of things in a hurry. Notice yourself rushing from one activity and task and meal to another. To support the practice of slowing down when you eat, play around with slowing down when you engage in other activities. Take your time and pay mindful attention to slowly brushing your teeth, driving your car, walking, or any other activity you do on a regular basis.

I practice slowing down when I do yoga. When I stand in the mountain posture (feet hip-width apart), I take a deep breath in as I raise my arms overhead, and, as I breathe out and bring my arms to my sides, I move them as slowly as I can. I feel the weight of my arms and feel gravity pulling them down. This one unhurried movement slows down my thoughts, my breath, and the rate at which I proceed. It is amazing how it helps me feel more calm, relaxed, and at peace. Try it now and see how you feel. Slowing down helps you savor your food and your life more fully.

How slow is slow enough? For starters, you might have heard it takes about twenty minutes for your brain to register fullness. That's correct and that's pretty bad news for most of us who have eaten a meal and long forgotten about it in twenty minutes. So, if you're not really paying attention, you will be way too full by the time the brain fully catches on. Slowing down can result in eating less because the awareness of fullness will help you stop.

If you are one of those naturally slow eaters, congratulations! You have this aspect of mindful eating under control. However, if you have a hunch that you are a speed eater, see if you can slow it down a notch or two. The habits you have developed around eating can be hard to break. You might not always take twenty minutes to eat your meal, but work at moving in that direction.

I—Investigate your hunger throughout the meal, particularly halfway through

BASIC INSTRUCTIONS: To be a mindful eater, it is important to be aware of your distractions and to keep bringing your attention back to eating, tasting, and assessing your hunger and satiety throughout the meal. In particular, if you bring an investigative awareness to your meal when you are halfway through, you may discover you are no longer hungry even though there is still food on your plate. You may discover you no longer find the food appealing. Give yourself permission to stop or to continue based on how hungry you are, not on old rules like "you need to clean your plate."

In addition to checking in with your hunger *before* you start eating, it is important to keep investigating your hunger *throughout your meal* so you can determine when to stop eating. Even if you find yourself rushing through your meal unaware, start embracing the idea that at least halfway through you will "STOP" and breathe. STOP stands for:

S—Stop when you're halfway through the meal

T—Take a breath

O—Observe the signs of satiety and taste

P—Proceed

When you are in the "observe" step, pay attention to your belly and note where you land on the hunger and satisfaction scale. If you feel satisfied, stop eating. If you're still hungry, continue eating. You can also ask yourself, *How does the food taste? Is the food worthy of my taste buds?* Or, *Am I only continuing to eat because the food is still there?* What you do next—continue eating or not—will be based on information from your body and your taste buds. This technique is a variation of one that has been used to help individuals successfully make appropriate responses in a wide variety of situations (Wise 2002).

Granted, this investigation of satiety and taste and using it to guide how much you eat is not as easy as it sounds. In fact, stopping eating at the point of "satisfied" rather than "full" is one of the greatest challenges for many of the people I teach. Two common questions arise:

"How do I know if I'm satisfied?" Right now you might get to "full" and completely skip over the "satisfied" feeling (which I describe as no longer feeling hungry) before you feel full. There will be a subtle cue from your body that says *enough*. Listen closely.

"Why do I keep eating, even though I'm satisfied?" Even when you notice being satisfied, you might still find it difficult to stop eating. Eating past the point of biological need or satisfaction happens for all kinds of reasons—some better than others. Here are the three most common reasons people tell me they eat more than they need:

"I love food and it tastes so good that I don't want to stop." If this is your experience, it can be helpful to remind yourself that this is not the last time you will have good food or be able to eat [fill in the blank]. In fact, part of the problem is that food is abundant and readily available. Don't worry. You will eat tasty food again. When you're satisfied, pack it away for later or throw it away (more on that strategy soon).

"I have a fear of being hungry." If you have been on diets in the past, the memory of being restricted in how much you eat can turn into obsessions about food and an aversion to feeling hungry. If you fall into this category, there is a way to stop being driven by the past. It starts with investigating how you feel in the present. Mindfully attend to the thoughts and effects of your past conditioning. Assure yourself that you can always have food when you want it. We will talk much more about working with thoughts and beliefs that lead to overeating, but at this point it is helpful to start a curious, kind investigation of what they are.

Not wanting to feel hungry might also stem from childhood experiences. For instance, did your mother or grandmother teach you to eat the minute you stepped into the house? Many of our parents grew up in a time when food was scarce. For them, feeling full is a sign of being okay and safe, and a sense of emptiness (hunger) is a source of anxiety and discomfort. Unknowingly, our loving caretakers might have passed on some pretty emotional and dysfunctional ways of experiencing hunger.

"I have to clean my plate because I don't want to be wasteful." Have you been told to clean your plate because there are starving children somewhere in the world? Do you think about how much money you're wasting if you don't eat all of your food? If you have either of these thoughts or both, you may be riddled with guilt about throwing food away, even if you're not hungry any more. Being driven by these thoughts into overeating is an unconscious behavior that helps no one—not even a starving child somewhere in the world.

Roberta said, "This 'don't waste food thing' is a big deal to me. It seems self-indulgent or something to look inward and try feeling when I've had enough and to stop eating at that point. It is not comfortable for me to do that. But, I know that my overconsumption of calories is not going to solve world hunger. I'm obese and have been for many years, so my way of thinking about this is obviously NOT working for me."

Whatever your reason for cleaning your plate, now is the time to rethink your strategy. You can give yourself less food, you can save food for later, and you can throw food away. You might have become conditioned to not do any of this for a multitude of reasons, but it is one of the most important changes to make as you journey down this path of mindful eating. Remember, your stomach is not a waste-basket. It's no more wasteful to throw food into your stomach that it doesn't need than it is to throw it away. As Roberta said, this might create some discomfort at first, but it is the place to start. Unless you bring to light the beliefs that are keeping you stuck, you can't move past them.

Eating and socializing go hand in hand. And when you're involved in conversation, it can be difficult to remember to check in with your belly. When you don't pay attention to your hunger throughout the meal because you're distracted by other people, a practice of checking in at least halfway through can be quite helpful. Let your attention move from listening to others to listening to your belly. Don't get so caught up in the conversation that you forget to be aware of getting full.

Eating out at a restaurant is another time when it is particularly important to investigate your hunger throughout the meal. You are in control of what you order but not how much food is presented to you. Remember, the chef at the restaurant didn't check in with your hunger when he decided how much to give you. And, portion sizes have dramatically increased over the past twenty years. For example, according to a National Institutes of Health (2013) report, a soda has grown from 6.5 ounces to 20 ounces, and a serving of French fries has grown from 2.4 ounces to 6.9 ounces. Plate sizes are much larger than they used to be. I notice this when I'm shopping at estate sales. Have you seen the tiny size of dinner plates from fifty years ago? To avoid falling prey to our current supersize mentality, try some new strategies. If you are eating out with someone else, share a meal instead of getting two. If you're alone, take the extra food home for later or throw it away when you're full. To help you stop, you can put your napkin over your food or ask the waiter to take the food away. If you know the portions are way too big, you can even tell the waiter to put half of the food in a takeout container before you get your meal.

Cheryl said, "I have described myself as a short woman with a man-sized appetite. Since investigating my hunger throughout the meal, I have found I have a petite appetite. I am astounded to learn I need to put less food on my plate to start the meal. Not out of deprivation, but because I've learned that *full* is not that far into the meal!"

Is it ever okay to eat past the point of satiety? Absolutely. It is reasonable to occasionally choose to eat more than you biologically need. For instance, when I go on vacation, I search for wonderful restaurants or specialty foods that I don't get to experience at home. I have eaten my way across many cities and countries, and when I consciously choose to eat more than I really need, I do so with absolutely no regrets or guilt.

On my birthday, my friend Ginny made me amazing homemade tamales and, while one would have left me satisfied, I ate two. Since Ginny was dying of bone cancer and nearing her final days, I knew I would not be able to share a meal like this with her again. The tamales were wonderful, and I mindfully and joyfully ate more than I really needed. I still have fond memories of that meal.

When to stop eating is determined with each meal and each circumstance. In general, stop or continue eating based on your biological hunger, not the amount of food on your plate or any other justifications you might come up with. You might feel satisfied halfway through, or you might discover that you're eating food you no longer want. Give yourself permission to stop or to continue based on a new mindful awareness of your actual hunger or fullness.

C—Chew your food thoroughly

BASIC INSTRUCTIONS: Pay attention to the multitude of sensations available to you as you chew your food. Notice the variety of tastes registered inside your mouth and whether you enjoy what you're eating. Notice what happens to the food as you chew. How long does it take to thoroughly chew your food before you swallow it? As you continue to chew and swallow, can you sense digestion beginning to occur and hunger beginning to dissipate? Chew each bite thoroughly before you move on to the next.

Learning to mindfully eat involves bringing your attention to the taste, smell, and sight of food and taking your time as you savor your food. However, in my experience, slowing down in order to appreciate all of these things is one of the greatest challenges we face as we learn to mindfully eat. How do you put "slow down" into practice in our fast-paced world? A simple way to support slowing down and mindfully eating is to bring your attention to chewing. Anything to which we bring our attention can become a meditation, and meditating on chewing can turn an ordinary process into an extraordinary experience.

Chewing can even make the difference between life and death. Lino Stanchich (1989) tells the tale of his father, who had been in prison camps during World War II. While in prison, Lino's father lived on a starvation diet of a daily bowl of soup consisting of potatoes and some other vegetable, and an occasional bit of meat. He intuitively experimented with keeping any precious food he received in his mouth for as long as possible and chewing—starting with fifty times a mouthful. He not only felt his thirst being quenched, but he also had more energy. His "magical number" of chews was 150, and the more he chewed, the more energy he had. At the end of the war, the only three men who survived of the thirty-two who were captured together were Lino's father and two others who had joined him in his practice of chewing. His account of how he survived, literally through chewing, became lifesaving advice for Lino when he himself was detained for two years in a prison camp in Yugoslavia.

My yoga teacher lived and taught yoga at the Kripalu Center for Yoga and Health in Massachusetts. He related the story of when Lino Stanchich came to do a "power eating" program there and encouraged people to chew each bite fifty times. At Kripalu, an institution that serves hundreds of meals each day, the kitchen staff keeps close track of how much food is consumed. Over the course of a week, the staff reported a drop in food consumption by one third when people were instructed to "power eat." Think about the consequences of reducing your food intake by one third.

Lino is not the only one telling us to chew thoroughly. Horace Fletcher, called "The Great Masticator," was one of the original health food enthusiasts of the Victorian era and even made it into our modern lexicon. Merriam-Webster's dictionary defines *fletcherism* as the practice of eating in small amounts and only when hungry and of chewing one's food thoroughly (Merriam-Webster.com, s.v. "fletcherism"). Fletcher's basic tenets were that "one should eat only when genuinely hungry and never when anxious, depressed or otherwise preoccupied; one may eat any food that appeals to the appetite; one should chew each mouthful of food thirty-two times or, ideally, until the food liquefies; one should enjoy one's food" (Merriam-Webster, Inc. 2011). Great advice then; great advice now!

Recently, researchers sought to test Fletcher's doctrine of chewing. They compared the difference in the impact of thirty-five versus ten chews per mouthful. They discovered that higher chewing counts reduced food intake despite increased chewing speed (Smit et al. 2011). Another study found that people who chewed their food forty times versus fifteen times ate fewer calories and had lower levels of the hormone ghrelin, which stimulates appetite, and higher levels of a hormone that reduces appetite (Li et al. 2011).

Why is chewing so important and powerful? Biologically, chewing your food activates many processes. Chewing breaks down food particles into smaller pieces upon which the digestive enzymes can act, lubricating and softening food so that it is more easily absorbed in the stomach and digested, lessening problems such as constipation and acid reflux. When food is in the mouth, the sense of taste is activated. This helps the body identify essential nutrients and harmful, potentially toxic compounds and process them accordingly. Your mouth acts like a food processor for your meal, allowing you to gain much greater nutritional value and more energy from your food. The act of chewing sends messages to the brain that help you register satiety, and saliva produced through chewing promotes healthy teeth (Pedersen et al. 2002). Finally, my favorite benefit from chewing thoroughly is that it helps you slow down and savor and enjoy the taste of your food.

Having tried to chew my food up to one hundred times, I will not be recommending that much chewing to you. It makes my jaws ache just thinking about it. However, I am suggesting you pay much more attention to chewing than you do currently and chew each bite thoroughly before swallowing. Don't overthink this or chew to the point where you're making the meal a miserable experience. This practice is not meant to ruin eating for you, but rather to enhance the taste of food and your health. Use the focus on chewing as a means for slowing down and savoring—which brings us to the last of the BASICS.

S—Savor your food

BASIC INSTRUCTIONS: Savoring your food means taking time to choose food that you really like and that would satisfy you right now—food that honors your taste buds and your body. Savoring your food happens when you are fully present for the experience of eating and the pleasure that it can bring. Your attention rests on the complete range of sensations available in each bite. If you really like it, experience the joy of savoring. If you can't savor it, why eat it?

The first part of "savor" is choosing food that you like and that would satisfy you. How do you choose the food you want to eat? Do you pause to reflect on the type of food or flavor that would satisfy you, or do you fall prey to the "see food, eat food" diet, eat when you're distracted, and eat out of habit? Taking time to consciously choose the food you want can help you feel more satisfied when you're done. For instance, if you have a desire for chocolate, do you let yourself have it? Or, do you tend to graze and eat all kinds of other foods until you finally give in and have the chocolate? No amount of celery, carrot sticks, or rice cakes can satisfy your desire for chocolate, if chocolate is what you want. Why not have what you want to begin with?

Studies have demonstrated that taste is truly acquired. If you are exposed to certain kinds of food over and over again, you will begin to prefer them. If you have been accustomed to eating highly refined foods with artificial flavors or foods with high amounts of sugar, refined salts, and certain types of fats, your taste buds have been dampened and habituated to prefer this way of eating. The good news is that if you trained your taste buds to want overly processed food, you can also train them back to sanity.

This transformation does not need to be forced. If you can mindfully eat fast food and really love it, by all means have it and savor it. In fact, many people just starting the mindful eating journey say they prefer to eat fast food or junk food instead of fresh fruits and vegetables. The proliferation of fast food restaurants and the junk food in every vending machine support that contention. However, I need to warn you that practicing with the concepts in this book has ruined fast food for many people. I don't tell anyone what to eat, but I ask them to really pay attention to how it tastes. Under the microscope of investigation, your taste buds mindfully rediscover their senses.

Rachel, a twenty-five-year-old graduate student, is one such convert. About a year into exploring mindful eating, she came to me one morning and said, "You're going to love this story. I tried to go to Burger King and get some food last night and everything tasted awful." Marilyn, a fifty-four-year-old woman trying to get her diabetes under control, said she was never going to give up doughnuts with maple-flavored icing. But, by the end of ten weeks, she reported having no appetite for the circle of fat with artificial flavoring and sugar on top. Personally, I was a four-can-a-day diet-soda drinker before I started practicing mindfulness, and I thought I really loved it. One month after my first meditation retreat, I was shocked at taking a sip and only tasting chemicals. My diet soda days were over.

Savoring your food is a whole-body experience, making eating a holistic endeavor. When you notice the effect of food on your body, lots of information can begin to flood into your awareness. Too much fat can make your stomach feel queasy. Overly processed food doesn't satisfy you for long or give you energy to last throughout the day. Sugar makes you feel famished and exhausted, and regularly eating the "crystal crack" messes with your body's ability to tell your brain you're full. Notice the next time you eat or drink something with a high sugar content and see if you experience the sugar crash about thirty minutes later. In contrast, notice the energy and vitality your body gets from fresh fruits and vegetables. Whole foods are processed more slowly in the body and sustain you through all of the demands of your day. Savor the food you're eating and notice how the body feels. Can you let this information guide what and how you eat?

The second part of savoring has to do with being fully present for your food and the pleasure it can bring. Bringing yourself fully into the present moment as you eat and savoring the taste can be all you need to reverse your unconscious approach to food. Let the taste of your food bring you back to the present. Be fully present for the taste. If the mind wanders away, bring it back. Use taste as a way of training yourself to be present. Return to the fresh, direct experience of taste over and over again.

At a workshop, I instructed people that we would be doing a mindful eating exercise with three kinds of chocolate. "There is something for everyone—milk chocolate with hazelnuts, dark chocolate with mint, and dark chocolate with cranberries and almonds. Come on up and get three pieces and then go back to your seat," I said. Peggy walked up to the table and picked out her chocolate. As she walked by me I saw her throw one of the pieces in her mouth and swallow it whole. "Wait! Wait!" I said. "We're going to eat the chocolate together as a group." A little embarrassed, Peggy laughed and got another piece. After eating the chocolate mindfully, Peggy reported that the piece she swallowed whole had no taste at all while the pieces she mindfully savored were nuanced with a multitude of flavors and brought great delight.

It is amazing to me that simply not paying attention can block the experience of taste. But when you engage in the practice of mindful eating, you regularly discover new information about your taste preferences and whether your body wants something or not. Be prepared to be surprised at what you discover when you become fully present.

You have at least three times a day when you can have a pleasant experience with food. Not that every meal will be a gourmet experience, but even simple foods can be delightful to the senses when you stop to pay attention. Savor your food. Enjoy the way it feels in your mouth and in your body. The whole experience can be delicious and delightful and free of guilt. Savoring mindfully, your relationship with food and your body begins to improve and your trust in your inner wisdom begins to grow.

MINDFUL EATING EXERCISES

Now is the time to take all of the BASICS of mindful eating and apply them to when you eat. The following instructions for mindfully eating a raisin and having a mindful meal or snack will get you started. While the exercises might seem a little formal or silly at first, try to put yourself into the mindset of discovery, exploration, and nonjudgment. Apply the attitudinal quality of mindfulness called "a beginner's mind." Having a beginner's mind—being able to see or taste something with curiosity and novelty—is necessary when learning something new. You could even pretend that this is the first time you've ever eaten.

The first eating exercise below, developed by Jon Kabat-Zinn (2013), is quite famous among people who teach mindfulness. It's sometimes called the "raisin meditation." I highly recommend doing the raisin meditation first and then applying what you learn as you follow the instructions for mindfully eating a meal or snack. At first you will want to do these exercises alone so you can focus your attention entirely on eating. In other words, turn off your cellphone and computer, put down your reading material, and eliminate any other distractions. After eating a few meals this way, you will find it easier to do in the company of others.

Exercise: Mindfully Eat Some Raisins

For this exercise you will need three raisins as well as paper and a pen to write down your experiences. You will explore the raisins through all of your senses—through the sense of sight, touch, smell, hearing, and taste. You can download an audio recording of this exercise at http://www.newharbinger.com/33278 or http://www.lynn rossy.com.

Start by placing all three raisins in the palm of your hand. Start to get a sense of the raisins, your thoughts about the raisins, and your thoughts about this exercise. As best you can, let everything go except your direct experience of the raisins.

Using the sense of sight, notice what they look like. Take your time and explore the raisins in detail as if you have never seen a raisin before. Don't be afraid to move them around in your hand. You might notice their irregular shape and size, their wrinkles, and how they shine in the light. How are they alike? How are they different? Take a few moments to examine the raisins with the sense of sight; and write down what you notice.

Next, move to the sense of touch. What do they feel like in the palm of your hand? Pick one up and notice what it feels like. What do those wrinkles feel like when you put a raisin in between your fingers? Notice the texture—is it squishy or sticky? Notice, through touch, what there is to be discovered, and write it down.

Now we'll move to the sense of smell. Pick up one of the raisins or bring the entire hand with all three raisins to your nose. What do you notice about the smell? You might have never smelled a raisin before. Sometimes people report that it smells "earthy" or like licorice or wine. See if one raisin smells more pungent than another. Write down what you notice.

Next we'll move to the sense of hearing. That might sound a little strange, but have you ever tried to hear a raisin? Try to be as open-minded as possible about your experience. Little children love doing things that are unfamiliar and different, yet as we grow older, notice how we tend to be "too old" to do something like this. Move the raisin back and forth between your fingers and see what you discover. Write down what you notice.

Finally we will move to the sense of taste. Ah! The sense you've been waiting for. But, before you put one in your mouth, take a moment to decide which one you want to taste first. Is it the big one? The little one? Notice what kind of preferences arise as you look at the raisins. Mindfully choose the first raisin you want to taste and place it between your fingers. Notice how easy it is for your fingers to reach your mouth. You could even close your eyes and that raisin would find your mouth.

But wait! Don't chew just yet. Simply place the raisin on your tongue and notice what the raisin feels like before you start to chew it. Move it around with your tongue; be aware of the increase in saliva oozing into the mouth in preparation for digestion. Notice the desire to chew. Notice any other thoughts you might be having about this exercise and just let them go. Come back to the direct sensation of the raisin in the mouth. And, when you're ready, beginning to chew.

Notice what it feels like to take that first bite. Slowly chewing the raisin and noticing what happens. Notice the taste, where different tastes are registered in the mouth, and how taste changes over time. Notice how the tongue gets involved in chewing the raisin. Chewing thoroughly before you swallow; and, after you swallow, notice what sensations are still evident in the mouth. Notice any desire to move on to the next raisin. Write down your experience of eating and tasting the first raisin before moving on to the next.

Repeat the exercise with the next two raisins, one at a time. Don't assume that every raisin will be the same. Stay open to the idea that they might be quite different from one another. Be fully present for the taste of each raisin.

What did you notice?

Write down any observations you had about the exercise. What did you notice about the raisins? How is this different from the way you normally eat? What was the experience like for you? You didn't have to like it or not like it. There is no right or wrong answer.

Don't let the fact that you don't have raisins in the house or that you absolutely hate raisins stop you from doing the exercise. The idea is to take three small pieces of food and bring your entire attention to assessing them, chewing them, tasting them, and swallowing them. Explore with different kinds of food—three dried cherries, three small bites of chocolate, three pieces of cantaloupe, or three blueberries.

Hopefully you wrote down your reflections as you did the exercise. Maybe they sound like some of these. Janet said, "I've never really tasted a raisin before or noticed the sweetness and flavor of one single raisin." Susan didn't like raisins but said, "It made me realize how fast I usually eat. I don't know why I eat so fast, but I always have. Maybe it's because I don't want people to watch me eat." Sally said, "The first thing I noticed was how much resistance I had to the exercise. I just wanted to get it over and get on with it. I didn't want to write down my reactions. I already had the second one in my mouth before I was finished with the first. This was very enlightening." Margaret said, "I thought I knew everything there was about slowing down and savoring my food, but I've never explored food like I did with those three raisins. It makes me very excited to see how I do when I apply that to eating a meal."

Although this exercise has been around for many years, recently researchers have examined the effect of mindfully eating a raisin on the degree of enjoyment people have when eating other foods. Participants were randomly assigned to one of three groups: a mindful raisin-eating group, a non-mindful raisin-eating group, and a no raisin group. Compared to the latter two groups, participants in the mindful raisin-eating group indicated significantly higher levels of enjoyment of other foods after doing the raisin exercise (Hong, Lishner, and Han 2014).

Now is your chance to take what you've learned from the raisin exercise and the BASICS of mindful eating and apply it to your eating at other times. The next time you eat a meal or snack, use the exercise below to guide you. This exercise borrows aspects of a mindful eating exercise used in MEAL (Mindful Eating and Living Program) and shared with me by Brian M. Shelley (Dalen et al. 2010).

Exercise: A Mindful Meal or Snack

Pick a time when you would normally eat a meal or a snack. You will be using all of the BASICS in order to determine hunger, choose and assess your food, slowly eat and savor, and stop when you are satisfied. As best you can, approach this eating exercise with mindful openness and curiosity. You can download an audio recording of this exercise at http://www.newharbinger.com/33278 or http://www.lynn rossy.com.

Before eating, bring awareness to your body and your breathing. Let your belly be soft and full. Take three full deep breaths. Let the breath relax you and help you settle into the present moment. Start by checking in to see how hungry you are. Use the Hunger and Satisfaction Scale to gauge your current state of hunger or fullness. Explore what hunger feels like in the belly, noticing its pleasant and unpleasant qualities. Notice the sensations that occur in the mouth and in the belly with the mere thought of eating.

If you haven't chosen food to eat yet, check in to see what would taste good right now. Can you get a sense of what the body would like to eat or what tastes would be pleasing to you? Once you have your food in front of you, take some time to assess it. What does it look like? What is the color and shape? Where did it come from? How nourishing do you think it is? What does it smell like? Acknowledge the importance of food for your body's health.

When you eat, can you take your time? You can slow down by chewing your food thoroughly and by putting down your fork or spoon between bites. Watch any distractions or thoughts, let them come and go. Keep coming back to the sensations involved in eating and tasting.

As you eat, notice whether you are enjoying the food or not. Focus on the sensations of taste—sweet, sour, salty, pungent. Keep coming back to the taste of your food. If you notice you aren't enjoying it, can you stop eating? If you enjoy it, how present are you for the pleasure of the experience? Savor your food.

Throughout the meal, noticing how your hunger level moves toward feeling satisfied. Particularly halfway through, stop and assess where your hunger level is again. If you're hungry, continue to eat. But, if you notice a sense of satisfaction, stop. Notice if it is difficult to stop at this point and inquire as to why. Give yourself permission to stop, even if there is some food left on the plate. If you normally would eat more, notice what it feels like to stop before complete fullness, exploring the pleasant and unpleasant aspects of this. Remind yourself that you can always have more later.

What thoughts and emotions are present as you eat and as you decide to stop? What beliefs and stories do you tell yourself about food and eating?

Be present for the last bite as fully as you were for the first bite. And if you eat more than enough, or feel too full, knowing that you have not blown it, but that you are simply now aware of this fullness. It takes time to learn new ways of eating and stopping. Every time that you eat is a time to practice again. Practice bringing kindness to yourself and curiosity to the practice of mindful eating.

What did you notice?

Which of the BASICS is the most difficult for you? Which is the easiest? How is this different from the way you normally eat? How will it change the way you eat in the future? Eating meals and snacks with the BASICS as your guide can help you begin to uncover your mindless eating habits. Awareness of your current habits is the first step toward changing them.

PRACTICING WITH THE BASICS

You can choose one of the BASICS to work with or work with them all at once. Follow them as best you can and as often as you can, knowing that there will be times when it will be next to impossible to eat this way. Write down the BASICS and put them on your computer, on your mirror, on the dining room table, or in the car; tattoo them on your hand (just kidding!) or put them wherever else you might see them on a regular basis. You might have never given these a second thought before, and finding ways to cue yourself to remember them can be helpful.

Eating mindfully requires the ability to focus, maintain your attention, and keep bringing your attention back to eating when you notice that your mind has wandered. Every meal might not get your full attention, but try to eat one meal or one snack mindfully every day. Even eating a few bites mindfully can help break the habit of mindless eating. Every time you eat can be a new discovery. Your consistent practice will reap benefits over time.

Learning how to become a mindful eater is a process—complete with its ups and downs. Rather than focusing on weight loss, the focus will be on how you feel and how food tastes, smells, and appeals to the senses. When you keep bringing your focus to your internal signals in a relaxed manner with kindness and compassion, you will learn many things about yourself and the food you eat. Your internal wisdom will guide you in the direction of health and well-being.

CHALLENGES:

- Becoming a mindful eater requires checking in with a part of your body you may have been avoiding for a while—your belly!

- Stress/emotional distress and physical hunger are often experienced in a similar way, and it can take some time to become adept at telling the difference between them.

- Food high in sugar, fat, or salt can set off biological cravings and can alter your taste buds—so they require careful attention as you begin to eat mindfully.

- Slowing down to pay attention to your food and its taste is a challenge in a culture operating on overdrive.

- You have spent a lifetime developing habits, ideas, and thoughts about food and eating. Understanding and changing them will take time and patience.

THE GOOD NEWS:

- The BASICS of mindful eating are a complete set of guidelines to help you become conscious about what, when, why, and how you eat.

- Breathing, something we do in every moment, is one of your best tools for understanding your hunger and your body. Take a deep breath now and feel the love!

- Your belly is your buddy and you can learn to trust its guidance.

- If you have trained your taste buds to want overly processed food, you can also train them back to sanity.

- Your body has a natural response to food that can guide you to greater health.

WHAT YOU CAN DO NOW:

- Regularly practice with the BASICS—using one at a time or all at once. If one is particularly challenging, practice with it for an extended period of time.

- Mindfully Eat Some Raisins: Use this exercise to help you learn how to use all of your senses when eating. You may want to experiment with different types of foods using the same instructions.

- A Mindful Meal or Snack: Do this exercise with as many of your meals as possible. Even eating a few bites mindfully during every meal can help break the habit of mindless eating.

CHAPTER 4

The Mindfulness Approach to Forbidden Food

This chapter introduces one of the key principles of intuitive eating: having permission to eat any kind of food you desire when you are hungry, otherwise known as "unconditional permission to eat." Based on this philosophy, you don't try to ignore your hunger signals, you don't classify food into acceptable ("good") and unacceptable ("bad") categories, and you don't generally attempt to avoid food considered bad—all things that you do when you're dieting (Tylka 2006). Abiding by this principle is an extremely important step as you learn to give up the diet mentality and make food your friend, but it often creates a tremendous amount of confusion.

What are your first reactions when you think about giving yourself unconditional permission to eat? Well, I'll tell you what I usually hear people say. "How can I eat everything I want, all of the time, and not get fat?" Or, "I'm terrified of letting myself eat what I want because I'll eat tons of junk food 24/7." What these statements demonstrate is the initial tendency to misinterpret the idea of having unconditional permission to eat. And, this misinterpretation is most likely a result of restricting and forbidding food in the past.

It's not surprising that the idea of allowing "forbidden" food causes anxiety, fear, and confusion. Forbidden foods can be a painful source of struggle and discontent. These are typically foods you binge on, overeat, and feel guilty about eating. Thinking about them rationally and trusting yourself to eat them sensibly might be hard to imagine. On the other hand, you might also sense a bit of delight in the prospect of allowing yourself a little more freedom with food.

FACING YOUR FORBIDDEN FOODS

Let's start our discussion about forbidden food with a review of the psychology of prohibition. What happens when you tell yourself you can't have something? You want it. Right? This is particularly true when it comes to food. As soon as you forbid yourself something, you want it more than ever. And, by golly, you eventually end up having it and oftentimes a LOT of it. These effects of dieting and restricting food are commonly described as the deprivation-binge cycle (Agras and Apple 2007).

Think about the last time you caved in and ate that gooey, sugary chocolate _____ [fill in the blank]. Here are some possible scenarios. You didn't just eat it, you binged on it because you told yourself you're *never* going to eat it again (or at least not for a *very* long time). You ate it extremely fast so you could pretend you didn't do it. You told yourself that if no one was looking, maybe the calories wouldn't count. Of course, they do count and you counted them and then you felt guilty. The guilt made you feel bad, so you said "screw it" and then you ate everything you'd been forbidding yourself and so the story goes. We have all been down this rabbit hole—probably numerous times.

The stress of eating (and then overeating) forbidden food can kick off biological cravings and dysfunctional thoughts and behaviors. At these times your ability to reason and make good decisions is significantly compromised. Your mind gets hijacked and you can't be expected to behave reasonably or eat sensibly. You binge because your rational, thinking mind is not available to help you.

The key to ending this pattern of depriving yourself and then overeating is to change your relationship to your food from one of prohibition and fear to one of allowing and safety. This is obviously easier said than done. The practice of mindfulness (being in the present moment with kindness and curiosity) supports you in humanely giving up the dichotomy of foods as good and bad.

Mindfulness allows you to relax and approach your forbidden foods with an ease that doesn't result in a binge. Mindfulness helps you assess, taste, and savor any food so that you enjoy every bite and stop when you are satisfied—not stuffed.

However, if you are just starting on the path of mindful eating, the journey of discovery that takes you to the land of peace with food can feel like a daunting adventure. A clear, comprehensive, and compassionate travel guide through the land of forbidden food can transform this journey into a wildly delightful trip. Although the BASICS of mindful eating are an absolute lifesaver when approaching forbidden food, to explore the entire terrain you will need to customize your own food travels on a daily basis.

As I sought to find a method for teaching the concept of unconditional permission to eat, I had an epiphany. It happened while musing with Denise, a graduate student who worked with me, about how to help people with this often difficult dilemma—"How can you allow previously forbidden food and not overeat?" She simply posed a question that a lot of other people ask me. "What do you do?" she asked. "How do you deal with the concept of unconditional permission to eat? You seem to have mastered this in your own life."

That's when the light bulb went off. I immediately thought of the crackers I had sitting in my lower left-hand drawer in my office. Crackers and I have a special relationship. When I'm at work in my office, I love to have something salty about 10:30 in the morning. I can't explain it, but I can set the clock by it. I'll be working at my computer and—wham—I need something salty. In the past, I would reach for the box in the food drawer and start popping crackers to get my salt fix. Because I was busy working on my computer (entranced with email, websites, and projects to complete), I'd forget to pay attention to what I was stuffing into my mouth until the box was empty.

I got my salt fix with the first couple of crackers, but I had no idea how much I was eating or when I'd had enough because I wasn't tuned in to my body at all. Around 11:00 a.m., I would stick my hand in the box to realize it was empty and regrettably feel the dead weight of crackers (lots of them) in my tummy. Come lunchtime, I wouldn't be hungry for a decent meal, would end up eating very little, and then would be hungry in the middle of the afternoon so I would snack on anything that happened to be around.

For a while I decided to forbid myself the irresistible crackers. At 10:30 a.m. I would still have my salt-and-cracker craving, but instead of crackers (which I no longer allowed in my food drawer), I would scramble around the office trying to find something to eat. You can ask my coworkers. Food isn't safe if I'm hungry. I ate stuff I didn't even want (chocolate, raisins, peanuts, power bars). But I really wanted crackers, and my body kept searching and eating and hoping to find the salty pleasure they would bring. Believe it or not, no amount of chocolate would satisfy my craving for crackers when it was crackers I wanted.

On my path to becoming a more mindful and intuitive eater, I decided to find a way to have my delicious crackers (previously forbidden) and not be so restrictive with myself. Before I went to work I decided to ask myself, *How many crackers would satisfy you at 10:30 a.m.?* At 7:00 a.m., my rational self was not interested in my demise, and I easily packed a reasonably sized baggy of crackers to take to work for my midmorning pleasure. I knew I only had a serving of crackers to eat. I could either eat them mindlessly and not get any pleasure from the experience, or I could eat them mindfully and really savor them. By allowing myself to have the crackers I wanted while acknowledging my habit of being overly engrossed in the computer at 10:30, this strategy helped train me to be more mindful about my food.

There were many times I would taste and savor the crackers but then completely space out until I realized there weren't many left. At this point, I would really pay attention. I'd type awhile and then I'd pause, eat a cracker and savor, type awhile, pause, eat a cracker and savor. This provided such good training that eventually I could bring the whole box of crackers back to work. At 10:30 a.m., I take a couple of handfuls out to eat and leave the rest.

When I examined the nuances and strategies associated with how I ate, I discovered it wasn't quite as simple as "no forbidden food." A more compassionate, understanding approach to having unconditional permission to eat needed to take into account the extremely embedded habits and triggers and subsequent cravings and binges that develop with food. Instead of forbidding myself crackers, I developed a strategy that taught me how much was reasonable to eat and gradually trained me to eat mindfully. I didn't get to the end (not overeating) without going through the middle and learning the lessons along the way. What resulted is a mindful approach to forbidden food called the Three Food Wisdoms.

THE THREE FOOD WISDOMS

The Three Food Wisdoms give you a less threatening way to think about forbidden food, one that honors the issues you discover as you overcome your anxiety with particular kinds of food. They infuse the practice of mindful attention, kindness, and compassion into the process in a very detailed way. Although they might seem paradoxical in nature, they represent a holistic approach for exploring the food you have previously denied yourself. They are:

Food Wisdom #1: Eating with permission (no forbidden food)

Food Wisdom #2: Eating the "right amount" (or "just enough")

Food Wisdom #3: Knowing and respecting your habits and triggers with food

Caveat: Sometimes I'm asked whether using Food Wisdoms #2 and #3 end up making you feel deprived and thereby diminish the concept of having unconditional permission to eat, to which I respond: If you don't have any difficulties with eating your forbidden food sensibly, then, by all means, don't worry about Food Wisdoms #2 and #3. However, if you are having difficulty introducing your forbidden foods without overeating, the Three Food Wisdoms are offered as extra guidance and support.

Food Wisdom #1: Eating with permission (no forbidden food)

What are forbidden foods? The first foods that come to mind are usually those high in sugar, fat, salt, and calories. These are foods you have determined are off-limits and "bad." You have overeaten them before due to their propensity for kicking off biological cravings, and you associate them with gaining weight.

Forbidden foods are *not* foods you have decided you don't want to eat anymore because of how they taste, how they make you feel when you eat them, or how they are processed. For instance, if you have truly discovered you don't like or want some kind of junk food or overly processed food, then it is not a forbidden food. Additionally, you may have come to peace with food you are allergic to and no longer want to subject your body to. In other words, you don't have to start eating Ho Hos (or food that makes you break out in hives) again if you have decided that you don't like how they taste, your taste buds like healthier snacks, or you have a wish to feel healthy.

If you don't think you forbid any foods, ask yourself whether you ever have any guilt when you eat. If you feel guilty or you criticize yourself when you eat it, then it is considered a forbidden food. Remember, the mind can be very clever. Take some time to explore how you talk to yourself about food and whether you have some secretly banned bounty. You can't overcome what you don't acknowledge.

Let's review the key issues to expect when you start giving yourself permission to eat. First of all, you may have a lack of trust in yourself. Food often becomes forbidden when you have overeaten it on numerous occasions and probably felt a lack of control. These experiences create a suspiciousness and fear of some types of food and a sense of failure as a person (someone without any willpower). Second, if you forbid food, you will crave it. Third, when you forbid food, you tend to idealize it—making it into something much more desirable than it really is.

As you reintroduce your forbidden foods, try to relax and enjoy the process. Bring an attitude of curiosity to eating food you might have avoided or denied yourself in the past. Don't be surprised if you feel a little out of balance. If you are afraid you won't stop eating, that is understandable. Regaining trust in yourself takes time. In fact, at first you may overeat your previously forbidden food. Forgive yourself if this happens. But don't give up. If you continue to let yourself know that anything is allowed, the urgency to have large quantities will eventually dissipate.

In fact, research shows that people can tire of eating the same kind of food—it's called habituation. Habituation is a decrease in response to a stimulus after repeated presentations (Heshmat 2011). The more accustomed you are to having something, the less novel it becomes and the less craving will you have. One caveat to remember, though, is that you need to be paying attention when you are eating or habituation will happen more slowly. When you eat your previously forbidden food, really pay attention, slow down, savor, and enjoy.

A wonderful story of habituation comes from Geneen Roth (2013), author of many books on emotional eating. She writes that when she first started on her path of healing from bingeing and dieting, she intentionally gave herself permission to eat chocolate chip cookies for two weeks straight—for every meal. She ate the dough raw. She ate them cooked. By the end of the two weeks she never wanted to see a chocolate chip cookie again. While this is an extreme strategy for overcoming the tendency to binge on a forbidden food, it clearly demonstrates the lengths to which you can go when you give yourself permission with food. She survived and lived to tell the tale of the no-longer-desired chocolate chip cookie.

Be particularly interested and curious about food that produces intense cravings. Having intense cravings for something probably means you are telling yourself you can't have it. You might have a desire for a pleasant experience (and an escape from boredom or some other difficult emotion), and you could find yourself obsessing about it. Memories of how wonderful it was in the past may flood your mind. This craving, caused by your thoughts, may make food sound even more delightful than it is.

As you begin to eat these revered foods, be aware of the difference between the actual taste and what you tell yourself about the food. When you eat your forbidden food mindfully, sometimes you will actually discover it doesn't taste that great. If it doesn't, stop eating it. For instance, this past Halloween I told myself that the candy corn someone left lying around at the office would be really great. However, one bite told me otherwise, and I threw out the handful I was ready to throw in my mouth. On the other hand, if you discover you still really like it, eat it and savor it. That is where the permission comes in. *You may have anything that you really want.* The trick is to eat it mindfully so that you can discover what it tastes like in the present—not when you were ten years old.

Keep being curious about your relationship to food and you will probably discover many layers of "forbidden." I thought I had traveled through my land of the forbidden when it occurred to me that cinnamon rolls were still lurking in the back of my mind with their tempting smell and cinnamon sweetness. Growing up, my mother made the world's best cinnamon rolls. We always had them on special occasions—particularly on Thanksgiving morning. My fingers would find themselves in the bowl of rising unbaked dough before Mom had a chance to make it into rolls. As a child, I ate cinnamon rolls without guilt and whenever the opportunity arose. As an adult, after my weight gain and subsequent dieting failures, cinnamon rolls became feared—the food to resist. If I ate one, I was afraid I would eat the whole pan. But I knew that I had to "get real" if I were to have any right to teach mindful, intuitive eating to others.

The cinnamon rolls that I feared the most were the Cinnabons! You know the ones. Those supersized monstrosities you smell at the airport as soon as you get through security—at least at the St. Louis airport. Cinnabon is right around the corner from the pat down. I had already overcome my fear of Snickers bars, French fries, chocolate milk shakes, and brownies. One day I decided I would face the mighty Cinnabon. Successfully through the X-ray machine (could they see my fear?), I made my way to the counter and bravely ordered my cinnamon roll. I refused to feel embarrassed, guilty, or any other self-deprecating emotion I might have felt for purchasing that many calories. Seven hundred thirty calories, to be exact, and 37 percent fat.

I would *not* feel guilty. I had the right to have any food I wanted. I relaxed and calmly gazed at my cinnamon roll and took the first glorious bite. Warm sugar, fat, and cinnamon. Wow! The first bite was pretty great. And, then, during the pause between the first and the second bite (I was mindfully eating, of course), I felt the rush of sugar in my body—similar to the rush I got many years ago when I experimented with drugs. Hmmm… this realization gave me pause. Okay, I took the second bite anyway. This taste wasn't as good and I could sense that I would be sick to my stomach if I continued to eat it. I got up and found the nearest waste can. I really didn't want any more, and the glisten of the cinnamon roll had been tarnished forever.

One at a time, the battle with forbidden foods can be met and overcome. The result is freedom. Not freedom to gorge yourself with all the food you want, but freedom to discover whether what you think you want is really appealing. If it is, eat it with pleasure. If it's not as good as you thought it would be, you can stop obsessing about it. Wouldn't it be nice to stop obsessing about the food you think you can't have?

Of course, there are always exceptions, and when it comes to food, the complexity of the issues are profoundly humbling. First, the no-forbidden-food philosophy is not meant to override medical advice you have been given by your health care provider about how to manage a medical condition that requires a certain diet. Mindfulness can help you understand and appreciate the reasons for these directives. Mainly, you will notice that when you eat certain foods, you get sick and sabotage your health. A compassionate, kind approach to your body—a mindful approach—would be to pay attention and be open to the right action for your body. What is the impact of eating food that is not recommended? What other foods can you learn to appreciate and enjoy that honor and respect your body? Instead of looking at the "don'ts" and reacting to them, can you find other types of food that bring you pleasure so you don't feel deprived?

Second, if you are introducing your forbidden foods when you feel emotional (e.g., sad, lonely, bored, stressed, anxious, angry), it will be more difficult to not overeat. Bingeing on food generally results from a combination of the content of the food (e.g., high in sugar, fat, or salt), negative self-talk, and your emotional state. We will talk much more about these topics later. Stay tuned! For now, try introducing your forbidden foods when you are in a relatively peaceful or relaxed mood.

Food Wisdom #2: Eating the "right amount" (or "just enough")

When you give yourself permission to eat anything you want, you will want to check in with your mind and your body. Breathe and belly check before you eat and reflect on what you are thinking about eating. Your mind might say, *I want two cheeseburgers with a big order of fries and a large chocolate milkshake!* However, if you drop below the neck and ask your belly how much it needs to consume to meet the body's nutritional and energy needs, you might hear a completely different answer. Order or portion out the amount of food you intuitively think your body is asking for, and in general don't eat more than that. Remember, you can always have it again later. There is no forbidden food.

In a culture where "Would you like that supersized?" was a popular advertising campaign, eating the "right amount" might take some training. Have you bought in to the idea that the more you get for your money, the better? This might make sense if you're buying nonperishable groceries, but it doesn't make sense when you're buying one meal. The fast food restaurant chains and mega food corporations capitalize on our fervor to get more for our money with their all-you-can-eat buffets and cheap products. You can certainly buy a lot for a little, but do you really want to and why? What you're buying along with the extra food are extra pounds you don't want or need.

From a historical perspective, although you might not have lived through the Great Depression, you are still affected by the consciousness of scarcity that developed during this period of time. The fear of not having enough food or money has rebounded into a need to have excess food and not waste anything because we might not have anything later. Despite the abundance of food and resources that many people have, these messages—get more for your money, don't waste, and eat a lot—have taken hold in our culture, and we are not the better for it. Don't get me wrong. I don't believe in being wasteful. And, I realize that many of us have to operate on a pretty tight budget. But when you buy more food than you need to begin with, eating all you can eat so you're not wasteful is not a sound solution.

We can learn a lot from cultures that have taken a different approach to eating. The Okinawans, renowned for their health, have heart disease rates and cancer rates 50 to 80 percent lower than Americans. They have a saying in their culture, *hara hachi bu*, which means eat only until you are 80 percent full. While most Americans eat until their stomachs feel full, Okinawans stop as soon as they no longer feel hunger. That's about 20 percent less food than we are used to consuming (Buettner 2008).

What does 80 percent full feel like and how will you know when you're there? Stopping eating when you are satisfied—no longer hungry but not yet full—can feel like a fairly elusive endeavor at first. Here are some suggestions that can help you eat the "right amount":

1. **Give up your membership in the "clean your plate" club.** Probably the biggest obstacle we face is our training, conditioning, and habit of eating until all of the food is gone. Given that portion sizes, plates, and bowls have grown dramatically over the past few years, this is particularly problematic. When we eat from larger containers, we eat more food. Physiological satiety cues are readily overridden by food cues such as large portions, easy access, and the sensory attractiveness of food. So in order to eat "just enough," you really have to pay attention to the internal cues to stop.

2. **Pay attention to how food tastes.** Being fully present for the flavors, smells, and tastes can satisfy you physically and emotionally. But, you can only enjoy and be satisfied with food you pay attention to eating. When you eat your previously forbidden food, you need to show up for the experience. On one hand, you will get to enjoy the food you have denied yourself for too long. (Personally, I'm thinking of a delicious chocolate flourless cake with raspberry sauce.) On the other hand, you might discover that some of the foods don't taste as good as you thought. The forbidden fast food

hamburger might surprisingly taste like cardboard when you eat it mindfully.

3. **Relax and slow down.** You don't have to rush through eating your forbidden food anymore. The signal that you have eaten "just enough" will be lost on you if you are racing through the experience. Slowing down will help you bring your mindful attention to this previously hurried activity. Take your time and savor.

4. **Ask your body.** Your body knows how much it needs before you start eating. Develop the habit of asking your intuitive self, *What is the right amount of this food for my body?* Portion out the amount of food you think you want before you start eating, and then don't go back for more. Brian Wansink (2006) indicates that when people pre-plate their food, they eat about 14 percent less than when they take smaller amounts and go back for seconds or thirds.

5. **Don't give up.** Don't be discouraged if you don't change your habit of overeating in one try. If you are accustomed to eating until you are full, it can take a while for you to retrain your stomach to feel comfortable with less food. Notice (with curiosity and kindness) each time you discover that you have eaten more than you wanted. Set the intention to pay more attention next time. But don't beat yourself up. This is a life-long journey.

As you begin to explore eating the "right amount" (or "just enough"), it is not uncommon to notice some anxiety when you stop eating before you are full. Simply be aware of any unpleasant feelings that might arise. You don't have to change the feeling, but acknowledge it with compassion. The act of pausing and examining the feeling of anxiety in the body and the thoughts that might be going through your mind can actually help reduce the discomfort and bring some sense of relief. Of course, taking a few deep breaths will also help you reduce those unpleasant jitters.

A willingness to be with a little bit of unease in the body can teach you a lot. Some of the anxiety might be from permitting food that was previously not safe. Some might be residual from the busyness of the rest of your day. When you rush around all day, you will bring the harried, frantic energy into the experience of eating. Stopping, pausing, breathing, and examining with curiosity will all serve to calm the anxious belly and mind. And, when you are calmer, the feeling of satiety can be more easily identified and acted upon.

Food Wisdom #3: Knowing and respecting your habits and triggers with food

As you learn to eat the "right amount" of your previously forbidden food, it can be helpful to season the process generously with kindness and compassion. You don't have to throw yourself into what feels like a minefield of forbidden food without taking into consideration the territory you have found dangerous in the past. Here are a few common habits and triggers that you might recognize. This list is by no means exhaustive, but it might get you thinking about how you unconsciously eat more than you need or want.

- You're distracted (lost in thought) and not paying attention to what you're eating.

- You eat while you're reading, watching TV, working on the computer, and so forth.

- You eat when you're stressed, angry, frustrated, or sad (emotional eating).

- You eat when you're bored—using food as entertainment.

- You eat by someone else's rules (e.g., clean your plate, don't waste food).

- You skip breakfast so you're ravenous later in the day.

- You finish your children's food.

- You drink alcohol on an empty stomach and then find yourself bingeing on food.

- You have junk food, candy, or other treats sitting around everywhere.

- You commonly eat straight out of the bag or box.

- You eat very fast (and maybe while no one's looking).

- You eat while you're driving in the car.

- You wait too long to eat and you're famished.

- You eat at night (maybe even sleep walking to the fridge!).

- You snack all day long.

- If you eat something you think you shouldn't have, you then eat everything in sight because "it's the last time you will ever eat this way again."

- You have certain types of food that you typically eat when you binge.

Even with mindfulness, the well-worn habits and hardwired triggers keep reappearing, and you might find yourself falling into their familiar routines. The road to mindfully making peace with food is filled with potholes. But you can learn to recognize when you've fallen into one, dust yourself off, and compassionately acknowledge your particular challenges when it comes to food.

It is helpful to recognize that you are constantly faced with food decisions. On some level, you are deciding whether or not to eat every time you see a food package or food item, go past a vending machine, walk through your kitchen, walk through the grocery store, drive down the street, fill up your car with gas, or see a fast food sign. Any of these environmental triggers can set off a pattern of overeating, and there are certain times you will be particularly susceptible to these suggestive cues. Think about how you behave around food when you're tired, starved, lonely, or stressed. Taking special care of yourself at these times by acknowledging how you feel can help you avoid turning to food for a fix.

One of the most common habits that often leads to mindless overeating is eating while you're watching television, reading a book, or working on the computer. Eliminating this habit or greatly reducing the time you spend doing it will help you be more in touch with yourself, your food, and your hunger. Of course, breaking the habit will take time, and at first you will probably feel some discomfort with "just eating." Notice the signs of withdrawal from multitasking. I even heard someone compare it to what people must feel like when they give up cocaine!

Once you identify your habits and triggers with food, it makes sense to make a plan for how you will deal with them. Ellen's real fear was pizza. Experience had taught her that no matter how many times she told herself she would eat only two pieces, before she knew it the whole pizza disappeared. She identified her habit of devouring the pizza while she watched TV.

Ellen used the Three Food Wisdoms to eat what she wanted and not get fat. This is what she did. Instead of eating at home in front of the TV, she found a pizza place that sells pizza by the slice. She bought one slice and found a quiet place in the restaurant away from the noise and the bustle. She sat down and paused for a moment while she took a few deep breaths. She assessed the pizza in front of her. Yes, she wanted it. She picked up the piece of pizza. As she closed her eyes, she took a bite and chewed it thoroughly. Bite by bite she did nothing else but taste and savor her pizza. At the end of the first piece, she checked in with her hunger. She was starting to feel satisfied but really wanted a second piece. She ate the second piece without guilt and thoroughly savored the experience. At the end, she checked in with her body. She felt satisfied and could stop. Right now she didn't need any more. She reminded herself that she could always come back for more pizza when she wanted it. Going forward, Ellen knew she could have her pizza and not overeat.

Now it's your turn. The next exercise will take you through seven steps for finding peace with your difficult foods. Right now, take a few deep cleansing breaths and feel your entire body breathing. Bring a sense of peace and calm to the following exercise as best you can. Whenever you feel anxiety arising, stop and take a few more breaths. Remind yourself that you are worth the time and energy you are giving to these exercises.

Exercise: Seven Steps to the Three Food Wisdoms

1. *Make a list of your forbidden foods that easily come to mind. You may always add more along the way as you become aware of them.*

2. *Make a list of your habits and triggers with food. After each one, list the alternate steps and strategies you will use. For instance, if you usually snack on something when you are reading, set the intention to either read or eat, but not both, particularly when you introduce forbidden food.*

3. *When you introduce a forbidden food, use the BASICS of mindful eating. Can you really binge on ice cream and chocolate brownies while you are breathing and checking in with your*

hunger, assessing your food, slowing down, investigating your hunger, chewing thoroughly, and savoring your food? Well, maybe. But, it would be a whole lot harder than if you were just scarfing it down.

4. *Decide ahead of time what you think would be the "right amount" of the forbidden food to eat in one sitting.*

5. *While you're eating your forbidden food mindfully, decide if you still like it or not. This may change over time, so stay tuned each time you eat it.*

6. *If feelings and thoughts of guilt arise, notice them and let them go. Eating food is a guilt-free experience from now on. Guilt only gives way to overeating.*

7. *If you overeat your forbidden food, don't judge yourself. Habits are hard to break.*

Keep working with your forbidden foods in this way until you don't have any left. Uncovering and making peace with the foods you have previously forbidden may take some time, or, once you get started, you might discover your ability to apply it quite globally to everything you eat. If there are some food items with which you feel completely out of control, leave them for later, when you feel a little more secure. You are not in an eating competition. You are on an eating journey. Be patient with yourself as you navigate your path.

Exercise: Body Loving-Kindness

To help you through the ups and downs of learning to mindfully eat and live, here are instructions for a formal mindfulness practice called Body Loving-Kindness. It is a powerful practice that inclines your heart and mind to open with kindness toward yourself. In this meditation, you are asked to offer yourself friendly wishes of peace, happiness, safety, health, and joy. However, there is no right or wrong way to feel as you do this exercise. You may feel kind and loving toward yourself. But, you may not. It might seem a little odd or even downright painful, particularly if you are used to saying more critical things to yourself (which, by the way, is true for everyone). The regular practice of saying nice things to yourself can, over time, begin to soften the hard edges of your judgment. When this happens you are more likely to treat yourself with kindness. You can download an audio recording of this exercise at http://www.newhar binger.com/33278 or http://www.lynnrossy.com.

> Start by finding a comfortable sitting position and bringing your attention to your body as a whole and the breath within the body. Notice how your body feels. Be aware of the sensations in your feet, the position of your legs, your arms and hands resting gently at your side or in your lap, the body sitting up in a regal, yet relaxed posture. Notice how your face feels and release any tension that you find. Then continue to scan the body from head to toe. Breathe out any tension that you find. After a moment or two, bring your attention to rest gently on the breath in the center of the chest. The heart center. Breathe in and out gently. Allow the breath to be soft and relaxed. Be fully present for the sensations that arise, exist, and pass at the heart center.
>
> Breathe gently in and out of this human heart. Breathe in and offer yourself the first phrase, "May I be peaceful," into the center of the chest—into the heart center. Gently breathe in "May I be peaceful" to the top of the head, to the tips of the fingers, to the soles of the feet. Take your time. Savor the words as you breathe them into your heart. "May I be peaceful."

Breathe gently in, and out of this heart, rest the second phrase, "May I be happy," in the center of the chest. Breathe it in and permeate the entire body with the wish to be happy. Sense the energy of the wish for happiness moving through your entire body. Feel the breath flowing in and out of the heart center. "May I be happy."

Breathe gently in and out of this human heart, this heart just as you find it. Rest the phrase "May I be safe from inner and outer harm" in the heart center. Breathe gently in and out. Let the wish for safety bathe all of the cells of your body. Fill your body with the wish to live free from harm. "May I be safe from inner and outer harm."

Sense this body just as it is. Breathe in and out of this heart center. Rest the phrase "May I be as healthy as I am capable of being." Rest this wish for health in the center of the chest. Breathe it in to the top of the head to the tips of the fingers to the bottoms of the feet. Fill this body with the wish to be healthy. "May I be as healthy as I am capable of being."

Keep bringing your attention back to rest on the breath in the center of the chest. The heart center. Rest the final phrase, "May I live with joy and ease," in this human heart. "May I live with joy and ease." Breathe in and out of this heart, suffuse this body with joy, and delight in this precious yet ordinary human life. Fill this body from top to bottom with this wish. "May I live with joy and ease."

"May I be peaceful. May I be happy. May I be safe from inner and outer harm. May I be as healthy as I am capable of being. And may I live with joy and ease."

Stay here as long as you'd like, and when you return to the normal activities of your day, take these wishes of kindness into the world.

This is an exercise you can sprinkle liberally throughout your day. You can repeat the phrases to yourself when you first wake up in the morning. Repeat the phrases to yourself while you're taking a shower, driving to work, waiting at the red light, before you answer the phone, in between activities, and while you're walking from place to place. Say them again as you fall asleep at night. And, if you wake up in the middle of the night and can't get back to sleep, say them again instead of listening to all of your worries. To help you remember them, consider posting them beside your computer, on the bathroom mirror, or on the fridge. I especially like to end all of my meditation practices with these phrases.

Don't forget to use some kindness as you introduce forbidden foods and when you eat more than you think you should. Instead of feeling guilty and beating yourself up, send yourself some love. Soften your heart with compassion toward yourself and acknowledge the challenge of changing old patterns of behavior. Send yourself some kindness because being human means we suffer sometimes. Becoming your own best friend is part of this journey.

It can be helpful to make the phrases your own. You might not like the phrases I've suggested, so play around with using words that resonate more with you. You can use just one phrase or all of them. There is no right way or wrong way to practice, and there is no right way or wrong way to feel when you say them.

While the exercise instructs you to offer yourself loving, kind wishes, don't hesitate to spread the wealth to others. As you walk about your day, you can send stealthy kind wishes to everyone you meet—those you know and those you don't know. The more that you train your mind in this way, the more the mind will naturally be kind.

CHALLENGES:

- Introducing forbidden foods can cause anxiety, fear, and confusion.

- Our forbidden foods are often high in sugar, fat, or salt, which can cause biological cravings and overeating.

- Our memories about food can set off about as many cravings (and binges) as the actual taste and content of the food.

- Stopping before you're full is not supported in this "supersize me" culture.

- Your habitual habits and triggers will need to be identified and addressed as you introduce forbidden foods.

THE GOOD NEWS:

- You can find peace with food by giving yourself permission to explore the world of food without guilt.

- Don't forget the BASICS. Mindfulness helps you assess, taste, and savor your forbidden food so you stop when you are satisfied—not stuffed.

- Your intuitive self knows how much food your body needs. Keep checking in with its wisdom as you portion out the food you want to eat.

- Habits and triggers with food can be addressed and overcome by listing them and thoughtfully developing new strategies.

- Talking to yourself with kindness can help you partner with the ups and downs of the journey with forbidden food.

WHAT YOU CAN DO NOW:

- The Three Food Wisdoms: Begin to introduce your forbidden foods with the supports given to you in this chapter. Keep using the BASICS of mindful eating, explore what it means to eat the "right amount," and acknowledge your habits and triggers with food.

- Body Loving-Kindness: Practice this meditation every day, even for a few minutes. You can do it while you're sitting or lying down. You can also remind yourself of the phrases throughout the day, no matter what you're doing. Offer yourself kindness (even if you don't always feel kind) and offer it to others. Notice what happens over time as you train the heart and mind in this way.

CHAPTER 5

Thoughts and Beliefs
That Lead You Straight
to the Fridge

L isten to the following dialogue inside Samantha's head.

Samantha One: Oh my! Doughnuts! Let me eat one fast so no one sees me. I know I shouldn't, but it would be SO good.

(Samantha quickly swallows the doughnut almost whole!)

Samantha Two: I can't believe you just ate that doughnut! Do you know how much sugar, fat, and carbs you just ate?! All you think about is food!

Samantha One: Well, if it wasn't in front of me I wouldn't have eaten it. It's not my fault. People at work always bring in bad food so there are too many temptations!

Samantha Two: You're never going to be able to lose weight. You will always be as big as a barn!

Samantha One: Oh yeah? Well, let me show you. I'll go back and eat as many doughnuts as I want. What do you think about that?!

In the process of making peace with food and yourself, it is important to be aware of and acknowledge the thoughts that are going through your head. Dialogues like this might go through your mind more often than you'd like to admit, with the resulting hurt, pain, and associated overeating. However, the truth about thoughts is that most of them are ideas we have been conditioned to believe, and most of them aren't true. The problem is that you listen to them as if they were true and seldom think about questioning them. When you think thoughts often enough, they become beliefs. Further, when you're not paying attention (which could be a lot of the time), these thoughts and beliefs run your life—often on a path straight to the fridge.

The field of psychology has come up with a term for these "untrue" thoughts and has labeled them cognitive distortions— errors in thinking we engage in automatically and habitually (Beck 1967; Burns 1980). The more you fall prey to these types of thoughts, the more likely you are to feel depressed, anxious, and stressed. Feeling distressed then results in self-defeating behaviors like overeating.

This chapter goes into great detail about thoughts. You'll get a chance to know yourself a little better as you uncover your own favorite (and dysfunctional) thinking patterns. You don't have to change your thoughts or fight with them. Instead of being dictated by them, you will learn how to pay attention to your thoughts with mindfulness, holding them in your awareness with kindness and curiosity.

Changing your relationship to thoughts will help you befriend them and yourself. As a result, you will be able to respond to thoughts and situations like the one above without spiraling out of control. You will learn to manage the thoughts and resulting beliefs instead of letting them hurt and manage you. Ultimately, you will be directed toward behaviors that support your desire to eat wisely sanely and live the life you want. "Watch your thoughts, they become words; watch your words, they become actions; watch your actions, they become habits; watch your habits, they become character; watch your character, for it becomes your destiny" (Swensen 2000, 115).

THOUGHTS THAT RULE OUR LIVES

How many thoughts do you think you have in a minute? It's been said that we have between thirty-five and forty-eight thoughts per minute (or 50,000 to 70,000 thoughts per day). Whether this is accurate or not, the main idea is that we think *a lot*. Thoughts are constantly popping up in our minds that are automatic, ruminative, repetitive, and predominately useless or negative. If you don't believe me, just stop for a minute and listen to what goes through your head. You will discover that you can't predict from minute to minute what your mind is going to say. You can only begin to recognize particular patterns. Sometimes I feel like my mind waits in anticipation for me to wake up in the morning so it can torture me with its usual nonsense.

After listening for many years to the stories of how people think when they struggle with food and their bodies, I constructed a list of cognitive distortions that are commonly reported (loosely based on Burns 1980). See if you recognize them and begin to notice when you engage in the following types of unhelpful thoughts:

- Categorizer (It's all-or-nothing, good and bad, right or wrong, and white or black)

- Rule Maker (I should, must, ought to, and have to)

- Perfectionist (I must strive to be perfect)

- Defeatist (I'll never be able to; I give up)

- Two Year Old (No! You can't tell me what to do!)

- Blamer (It's his/her fault or It's all *my* fault)

- Comparer (I'm not as good as, less than, or worse than him/her)

- Labeler (I'm fat as a cow; my belly is disgusting; my thighs are wiggly)

The Categorizer

The *Categorizer*, who engages in "all-or-nothing" thinking, is alive and well in most of us, but is particularly active in the minds of people who struggle with how to make sense of their food and bring kindness to their bodies. When this thinking prevails, there is a tendency to put everything into a distinct category on one side or the other. Thinking in this way is why "unconditional permission to eat" is often translated into *I can eat everything I want, and as much as I want, all of the time.* It is exemplified by thoughts like *that food is bad* or *I can never have chocolate.* These types of thoughts are conditioned by the dieting mentality. Listen for the words *everything, always, never, good, bad, right,* or *wrong.* They are signs that you are engaging in the dichotomous thinking of a Categorizer.

The Rule Maker

From "all-or-nothing," you can quickly fall into the role of *Rule Maker. I shouldn't eat that because it has too many carbs* or *I should only eat salads at lunch. I should be a size 8* or *I shouldn't have such a big butt.* Just the word *should* implies that you are supposed to, but you don't really want to or it's impossible. It can feel like there is someone standing over you giving you rules you can't really live up to. Besides your own dictates, you are constantly barraged with other rules about what you should and shouldn't eat and how you should and shouldn't look. These voices develop from what you see on TV, in the movies, and in magazines. They are embedded in popular culture and consumer marketing that says you need to be something other than what you are. Even skinny people can't live up to the expectations surrounding us. Under conditions of perpetual discontent, you will feel incapable of getting it right. Listen for the voice that sounds like a scolding parental figure.

The Perfectionist

The Rule Maker sets the stage for the *Perfectionist*. Ah, this is one of my favorites because I practiced it quite a bit! The Perfectionist says that you have to do it perfectly. There can be no mistakes (only failures), and life is not okay by any standard less than the highest. If you are not perfect, you are not good. Under the Perfectionist's influence, you push yourself to the brink and still never feel satisfied. If you reach a dieting or weight goal, then you set a harder goal to achieve. If you have a Perfectionist inside your head, you know how it sucks the joy out of every aspect of life. Listen for the voice that sets unrealistic standards for you and your behavior.

The Defeatist

This brings us to the *Defeatist*. If you can't be perfect, why try? This pattern of thinking includes a combination of self-judgment (*I'm not capable of eating like a normal person*) and discouragement (*I've tried and failed! I give up! I might as well let myself go. What's the point?*). Thinking this way is a result of having too strict standards and believing you've never succeeded. Listen for the whisper of statements like *you're a loser* and *why try?*

The Two Year Old

A more rebellious, obstinate version of the Defeatist comes in the form of the *Two Year Old*. In the world of food and eating, the Two Year Old is rebelling against all of the other voices that have been telling her what to do for years. She often sounds like this: *Oh yeah? I'll show you. I can eat whatever I want and lots of it! Who do you think you are?* This voice is quite common when you have lived too long under the reign of the Categorizer, Rule Maker, or Perfectionist. Listen for the voice that leads you to sabotage yourself while feeling less than adult.

The Blamer

At this point it can be very easy to fall into being the *Blamer*. You blame your husband for watching everything you eat and making comments about it. You blame your coworkers for bringing in too much candy and cake. You blame the restaurant for giving you too much food. You blame the media for portraying pictures of skinny, anorexic models and actresses as the ideal shape and size. You blame your mother. Now there's a good one. Let's blame Mom for making you clean your plate when you were young or making comments about your weight. On the other hand, you might fall into blaming yourself for things that aren't even your fault. You might have inherited your mother's "big bones" or your father's "large nose." Instead of embracing your genetic inheritance, you belittle yourself for body shapes and sizes that are part of your lineage. Listen for the voice that wants to blame someone, anyone, for how things are. Note: If you have had people say hurtful, judgmental things to you in the past, I'm not condoning that behavior. To take control of your life, however, you must not let what other people say determine how you feel and what you do.

The Comparer

When you are the *Comparer*, you might hear yourself saying *I'm not as good as* _____ or *I'm better than* _____ . Either one is a setup. If you are in the mindset to deem yourself either better or worse you will be setting yourself up to eventually fail. Comparing yourself to others is a common fallacy. You usually focus in on the part of your body you like the least and compare it to the same part on others everywhere you go. For instance, I used to compare my thighs to everyone else's. I developed the belief that I needed to have a gap between my thighs, and I envied every girl who had one. If you had a "thigh gap" you were obviously much better than me. (By the way, I later discovered they are photo-shopped onto models if they don't have one already!) I wouldn't even date men who had smaller thighs than me! Listen for the voice that compares you to anyone else (known or unknown).

The Labeler

Last, but not least, is the *Labeler*. This voice sums you up in a neat tidy package that is often based on a quality you don't like about yourself. For instance, if you don't like your weight, you might say, *I'm as big as a barn* or, *I'm a fat cow*. If you haven't been able to stay on a diet in the past, you might say, *I'm a loser*. You can label your behavior or you can label your body as "ugly" and even "repulsive." These global negative judgments mislabel you and prevent you from seeing yourself with any kindness, compassion, or clarity. Self-criticism and judgment are epidemic in our culture. Listen for the judgmental labeling of yourself, in whole or in part.

All of the thinking patterns listed above give you a distorted view of yourself, produce incorrect beliefs, and lead to disordered eating. To make things worse, if you have disordered eating patterns, you might be prone to spending an inordinate amount of time thinking about food, eating, weight, shape, and related matters (Gleaves et al. 2000). Thinking a lot about food has its own consequences. Merely thinking about eating a forbidden food increases people's estimate of their shape or weight, elicits a perception of moral wrongdoing, and makes people feel fat (Shafran et al. 2010).

SOME WISDOM ABOUT THOUGHTS

Just thinking a thought, even if it isn't true, will have an impact for better or worse. Further, once you start thinking a certain type of thought, you are more likely to keep thinking it. Thoughts are laid down like railroad tracks in your mind. Once you've criticized yourself fifty times, a neural pathway gets created in the brain that will trigger criticism in a moment's notice. The more you practice judging, labeling, or any of the other thought patterns listed above, the more you will hear them on a regular basis.

The main thing to remember is that *thoughts aren't facts*—even the ones that tell you they are. That's right, thoughts are just conditioned ways of seeing and experiencing the world that develop over time. It is estimated that we might think "facts" two percent of the time. The other ninety-eight percent of the time, your thinking comprises beliefs, ideas, opinions, perceptions, and prejudices. This means you can choose to change how you relate to your thoughts by bringing your attention to them and working with them in specific ways.

Believe it or not, the voices in your head are trying to be helpful. They do not mean to harm, even when they sound mean and are misguided. For instance, the Perfectionist and the Rule Maker are trying to help you to achieve a certain goal or behave a certain way because they think that is what will make you happy. These thought patterns started to develop at a very early age when you didn't know any better and didn't have a lot of other skills for getting what you needed. However, as an adult, you can easily see that listening to these thoughts as if they are true is very hurtful.

WAYS OF WORKING WITH THOUGHTS

The good news is that you can learn to relate to thoughts in a way that buffers you from their fatal sting and ends their control of you and your behavior. The thoughts in your head can change from moment to moment, and each person's stories may sound different in content and characters, but the way we get caught up by them and how we release and let go of them is exactly the same.

Mindfulness of Thoughts

One of the most effective ways to work with thoughts is through the practice of mindfulness. When you use mindfulness, you are bringing a kind, nonjudgmental attention to whatever thought arises in your mind. It doesn't matter what the thought says or whether you believe it or not. You are not trying to get rid of thoughts or change the thoughts. It doesn't matter if you like or dislike them. Nonjudgmental awareness of the thoughts is what will give you freedom from them while teaching you to dis-identify with the thoughts—in other words, to no longer believe that they reflect who you are.

When you use mindfulness, or metacognitive awareness of your thoughts, you are not caught in the story line. To get an idea of what this is like, imagine that you are sitting at the edge of a small stream in the mountains and you're watching as each fallen leaf floats by in the water. You don't try to catch the leaves with a stick, but you let them flow by you unimpeded. Now imagine your thoughts are just like the leaves flowing downstream. They easily float by if you don't try to catch them. Or you can imagine your thoughts are like clouds that pass across the sky. They come and go, fade in and out, but you are just watching and being aware of them without needing them to be any different than they are.

For instance, if Samantha had been aware of the thought *Oh my! Doughnuts! Let me eat one fast so no one sees me*, she could have stopped, checked in with her belly to see if she was hungry, and then decided if a doughnut was what she really wanted. Just because a thought tells you to do something doesn't mean you have to obey. When Samantha heard the thought *I will always be as big as a barn*, she could have been aware of it with kindness and acknowledged the pattern of thinking as "categorizing" and "labeling."

An important step in having freedom from your thoughts is to realize how much grief they cause you. While it is impossible to suppress them (in fact, that often makes them worse), it is possible to be aware of your thoughts and to notice their impact so that you eventually become disenchanted with them. How helpful are the voices telling you terrible things? What have they accomplished, besides making you feel bad?

Through the practice of being with thoughts as *just thoughts, not facts*, you can be aware of them without reacting. Befriending your thoughts lets you get up close and be curious about them without being affected by them. Where did they come from? What do they feel like in the body? It can be quite enlightening to take some time to listen nonjudgmentally to your thoughts every day. To get better at this, it will be useful to practice mindfulness of thoughts during a sitting meditation exercise, which you will see at the end of this chapter.

Mindfulness of the Present Moment

When you are caught in your head—obsessing, worrying, planning, regretting, and all the other types of stories you engage in—you are not interacting with your life as it is in this moment. In fact, you've created a new reality that only exists in your head, and you're living out the fantasy while your real life passes you by. Things that stress us tend to loop in our heads over and over and until we "figure them out" or get distracted by something else. If you find yourself thinking about food, your body, or anything else in an obsessive, ruminative way, you can use mindfulness to bring yourself back to the present.

Ask yourself, *What is actually going on now? What does my body feel like? Is there tension? What does the breath feel like? What sounds are present? What do I see around me? What am I doing?* When you bring your attention to what is actually going on in this moment instead of being lost in the story in your head, life becomes manageable, if not enjoyable.

Eckhart Tolle, the author of *Practicing the Power of Now*, says, "As soon as you honor the present moment, all unhappiness and struggle dissolve, and life begins to flow with joy and ease" (Tolle 2001, 43). This might take some practice, but keep dropping fully, with gentle acceptance, into the direct experience of the present. Freedom from negative thoughts exists in this full, open-hearted awareness of now.

The Sky Is Blue

This next technique is from meditation teacher Joseph Goldstein, who developed it as he worked on his own difficulties with judgmental thoughts. The idea is this. When you notice negative thoughts arising in your mind, just tack on the phrase "the sky is blue" to the end of each judgment (Goldstein 2003). For instance, *my belly is huge—and the sky is blue. I can't believe I ate that whole plate of pasta—and the sky is blue.* Adding the neutral phrase after a judgmental one is a way of neutralizing the negative thought. They are both "just thoughts," and neither has to produce any more or less emotional impact.

Jessica said that she put "the sky is blue" after all of her negative thoughts for a week. It made her realize how many negative thoughts she had, and it shifted her focus from the negative thought to the absurdity of the inserted thought. Try it for yourself. Add "the sky is blue" after every negative thought that you have, even for a day, and notice the impact.

Is It True?

Since cognitive distortions are always errors in thinking, it is useful to question them so they don't get away with torturing you. When you notice a negative thought, ask yourself the question *Is it true?* You might hear *Yes, of course it is.* Then you need to take some advice from Byron Katie (2003), author of *Loving What Is*, and ask yourself one of her favorite questions: *Is it absolutely, 100 percent true?* There is hardly a thought that can pass the 100-percent-true investigation. The third question is the obvious next step. Ask yourself, *What's another way of looking at this?* There is always another way of looking at something. In fact, there are many ways of looking at everything. Unless you are used to thinking in mathematical equations or scientific calculations, almost everything is just a matter of opinion.

Respond to Your Cognitive Distortions

It can be helpful to respond to your cognitive distortions by answering them. Here are some different ways of responding to each cognitive distortion listed at the beginning of the chapter:

- To the Categorizer: Life cannot be measured out into all-or-nothing, white and black categories. Life is very gray and "right" is relative.

- To the Rule Maker: I can make up my own mind instead of listening to your prescribed "rules."

- To the Perfectionist: Nothing is "perfect" and that's okay.

- The Defeatist: I am worth the effort, no matter what has happened in the past.

- To the Two Year Old: I can act like an adult and do what feels right for me today.

- To the Blamer: I will take responsibility for what I want and need in the present.

- To the Comparer: I am incomparable and wonderful just as I am.

- To the Labeler: There is no label that can capture who I am as a whole person.

Of course, you can develop responses that resonate with you. After spending some time examining your thoughts, you will identify your favorite distortions and ways of working with them. Breaking their spell is a positive step in overcoming their influence.

Special Circumstances

When you are tired, lonely, sad, mad, or otherwise distressed, you need to be on high alert for negative thoughts. These are times when you are most likely to turn to food and turn a bad day into an even worse disaster, complete with a big eating fest. The next chapter will address methods for working with these challenging times and difficult emotions without using food. For now, be on the lookout for negative thoughts that go hand in hand with vulnerable feelings and extra trips to the fridge.

CULTIVATING HELPFUL THOUGHTS

In addition to changing your relationship with thoughts using the techniques listed above, you can also work at cultivating thoughts that are more helpful and nourishing to you. Just think for a moment about how you feel when someone says positive, encouraging comments to you. Then think about how you feel when someone directs negative, judgmental comments toward you. Generally, when you are complimented, you feel uplifted, and when you are criticized, you feel shut down. The same model applies when you are talking to yourself. When you understand that everything you think or say has an effect on you (for better or worse), then you will naturally want to think and say things that lead to positive results.

To help you see how important it is to consider the impact of your self-talk, get a paper and pen and do the following eye-opening exercise developed by Debora Burgard and found on her Body Positive website (http://www.bodypositive.com/yourbody.htm).

First of all, think of a negative statement (an "old tape") that you typically say to yourself, and write it down. For instance, I have often said, My thighs are flabby. Now imagine that someone said your negative statement back to you. For instance, someone might say to me, "Your thighs are flabby." Write down how it would make you feel to have your negative statement reflected back to you. When I do this exercise in the classes I teach, I have people sit in twos and whisper to each other. There is definite discomfort (and quite a bit of giggling) when I first ask people to do this. Some actually refuse to whisper the negative statement to their partner. They can't imagine saying something this horrible to someone else even though they talk to themselves like this all of the time.

The second part of the exercise is to come up with a thought that is the opposite of the old tape—something glowingly positive— and write it down. For instance, I would write, "My thighs are athletic, toned, strong, and beautiful." Imagine what it would feel like to have someone say your glowingly positive statement to you, and write that down as well. Would you feel good? Would you believe it or discount it?

Next, think of a thought that would be descriptively true, as if you are explaining what you see to someone who can't see, and write it down. This statement would not be loaded with either good or bad associations. For instance, I would write, "My thighs are in between my pelvis and my knees, and they are strong enough to help me walk everywhere I need to go." Now imagine someone saying the descriptively true statement to you, and write down how you feel hearing it.

Which statement feels better to you? The negative, the glowingly positive, or the descriptive? You don't need to be "glowingly positive" toward yourself because that may not feel honest, but you also do not need to be glaringly negative. Neither one is particularly helpful. Since you make up the things that you tell yourself, you can change your self-talk so that it is more objective and even supportive and kind.

However, in order to begin to change years of negative conditioning, it could be useful to make some unexpected and startling statements that break you out of your spell of negativity and unworthiness. Personally, I find humor to be particularly suitable for lightening the heaviness of the harsh judgments we inflict upon ourselves as well as the difficulties that we will ultimately face in life.

While struggling with my body image, I developed a strategy for changing my negative body talk by telling myself, *Oh my God! You're gorgeous!* every time I looked in the mirror. You know how your eyes go straight to the part of the body you don't like? The second that happens, look yourself straight in the eye and say something outrageous. It might seem funny, stupid, and even unbelievable, but really camp it up. The more theatrical, the better. If you laugh, you will feel better, and when you feel better you will be less likely to continue your negative battle with yourself. Try it for a while and see what happens.

If you have trouble with this exercise, you can work your way up to the overall "You're gorgeous" comment by starting with one part at a time. Move your attention away from a part of your body you tend to judge to parts of your body that you already appreciate. For instance, instead of judging your thighs, you could say, *I have amazingly thick, luscious hair!* or *I have strong fingernails that other women would kill for!* Don't be afraid to fake it before you make it.

WHAT DO YOU BELIEVE?

Your relationship with yourself is the most important (and longest) relationship that you will ever have with anyone. Now is the time to cultivate the type of relationship that mirrors the respect you are developing toward yourself. It starts with your words. Your thoughts and words become the actions you take and the habits you develop. Over time, those habits begin to harden into who you think you are. But, with mindful attention, they do not have to become your destiny.

How we talk to ourselves starts with what we are taught as children. You were invariably taught and learned to believe (consciously or unconsciously) many things about yourself that you heard from your parents, your siblings, your peers, and the culture around you. Some of these beliefs are supportive, and it is useful to acknowledge and hold on to these. Other beliefs deplete you and have diminished your ability to express your highest desires for your life.

I incorporated many beliefs that had an impact on me throughout my life: be a good girl, work hard, don't have too much fun, clean your plate, work hard (didn't I already say that?), be humble, be independent, don't ask for help, don't be loud (that one didn't stick!), finish your pie, and you're "just a girl." Almost all of these beliefs have an "up" side and a "down" side. For example, "work hard" has helped me get a lot of stuff done, but it also drove me to be a neurotic perfectionist.

Think about your own personal stories, life circumstances, and major decisions that have shaped your life. What was the impact of your childhood experiences—the kinds of foods you were fed, the messages you were given, and the models you had for how to be in the world? What has been supportive? What has been depleting? Which thoughts and beliefs do you want to hold on to and which do you want to let go of? Take some time, if you'd like, and journal your answers to these questions.

Learning to accept and respect your body and your life starts with how you talk to yourself and the beliefs you choose to guide you. When you say encouraging, respectful things to yourself, your body and mind will respond with more positive actions. Your beliefs will pave the way or put up roadblocks on your path. When you realize *Oh! Someone cares. And it's me,* you will be more likely to treat yourself well—feeding yourself nourishing food and moving your body in ways that feel delicious.

Exercise: Mindfulness of Thoughts

This meditation will illuminate your thoughts in an environment of exploration. Noticing the thoughts without judgment or striving to change, avoid, fight, or struggle with what arises. This practice teaches you not to be affected by the thoughts, but to befriend them with kindness. Do the following exercise for ten minutes, if possible, to learn more about your mind and how to cultivate a better relationship with it. You can download an audio recording of this exercise at http://www.newharbinger.com/33278 or http://www.lynnrossy .com.

Start by sitting for a few moments as you settle into an erect, yet relaxed posture. Let your eyes close or simply lower your gaze to the ground as you take your attention to your body and your breath. Briefly scan the body from head to toe and see if you can soften and release any tension you might find. Take a couple of deep breaths to help you relax and settle into this moment—into your body and into your breath. Then, settle into the natural rhythm of your breath. No need to control the breath in any way. It might be deep or shallow. Let the breath breathe itself.

To stabilize the mind, it is helpful to use the breath as the object of meditation. The breath is available as an anchor to the present moment. Simply know when you're breathing in and know when you are breathing out. Not thinking about the breath, but wordlessly experiencing the movement of the belly and chest in response to the breath.

It won't be long before you notice the mind has wandered—to a bodily sensation, a sound, or most likely to a thought. Simply notice and bring your attention back to the breath. We easily get lost in thoughts during meditation practice. It happens to everyone, every time. This is not a problem. When you notice that your mind has wandered to a thought, be aware of what you are thinking and then firmly and gently bring your attention back to the breath.

In order to become familiar with the thoughts you commonly experience, when they occur, you can use a soft label for them such as "worrying," "planning," or "judging." You might notice one of the cognitive distortions—Categorizer, Rule Maker, Perfectionist, Defeatist, Two Year Old, Blamer, Comparer, or Labeler. No thought is "good" or "bad." They are just thoughts, not facts. Notice them with kindness and curiosity.

You can imagine that your thoughts are like clouds passing across the open expanse of the sky. Or you might see pictures or visual images instead of thinking thoughts. If you see images, let them pass across your awareness like a scene from a movie. Once you've noticed that you are lost in a story, bring your attention back to the breath. All kinds of thoughts and images might occur to you. Not making any of them special or extraordinary.

Stay with the breath until your mind wanders. When it wanders, notice and label what kind of story you get pulled into. Then, without judgment, gently return your attention to the breath. Do this for ten minutes, if possible.

What did you notice?

It can be helpful to write down your favorite cognitive distortions so you can be on the lookout for them. Do not be alarmed by the thoughts in your head. They truly have no power except the power that you give them. Your thoughts are conditioned by the amount of time you give them and your reactions to them. Notice how negative thought patterns pull your energy down. Notice what happens when you release them and bring your attention back to the breath.

I told you I used to have extremely critical, judgment thoughts when I first started meditation practice, and I felt horrible about it. Over time, as I learned to accept the thoughts as "just thoughts" and let them be, I became inoculated against their negativity. I actually named my critical voice Betty and made friends with her. When she shows up, I invite her to sit down beside me and have a cup of tea. We are great friends these days and she doesn't get to run the show.

Practicing awareness of thoughts on a daily basis with a formal mindfulness exercise can change how you are affected by them. By sitting and watching your thoughts with kindness and curiosity, you don't suffer because of their content. And cultivating thoughts that are more productive or positive energizes you toward healthy actions instead of trips to the fridge. You are moving from the old model of listening and reacting to negative voices to the new model of watching thoughts pass through your mind, establishing healthier beliefs about eating and your body, and talking to yourself like you would to your best friend.

CHALLENGES:

- We mistakenly believe the obsessive, ruminative thoughts that run through our minds by the thousands.

- Cognitive distortions (errors in thinking) can contribute to feelings of sadness, worry, doubt, and being overwhelmed—feelings that lead us straight to the fridge.

- Try as we might, it is hard to not be affected by the constant conditioning from magazines, TV, movies, and music videos that reinforce an "only thin is beautiful" diet mentality.

- Our childhoods were rife with messages we incorporated into beliefs that run our lives—sometimes for the worse.

- Our minds are unruly and difficult until we train them to be different or train ourselves to respond to them differently.

THE GOOD NEWS:

- Most thoughts aren't facts, even the ones that tell you they are.

- You can learn to relate to your thoughts in ways that inoculate you against any negative effect.

- Fully experiencing and accepting the present moment can give you freedom from negative thoughts and errors in thinking.

- You can learn to examine and challenge your cognitive distortions.

- You can cultivate kind, inspiring, and helpful self-talk that encourages kind, inspiring, and helpful behavior.

WHAT YOU CAN DO NOW:

- Regularly examine your thoughts for distortions. Discover your top three thinking patterns using the labels in this chapter or making up your own names that better describe them for you.

- Work with your thoughts using the following methods: Mindfulness of Thoughts, Mindfulness of the Present Moment, The Sky is Blue, Is It True?, and Respond to Your Distortions.

- Mindfulness of Thoughts: Practice this meditation every day, even for a few minutes. Consistency of practice is more important than length of practice. Don't underestimate the ability of this formal exercise to dramatically change your relationship to thoughts.

CHAPTER 6

What Are You Really, Really, Really Hungry For?

Up until now, I've asked you to listen to your biological hunger and satiety signals. I've asked you to listen to your automatic, conditioned thoughts. You are now ready to examine some of the deeper issues that arise with eating, requiring you to listen and respond to the fluctuation of your emotions in ways that will support your health and well-being.

It is quite common for people to use food as a fix for everything from a little anxiety to a disappointing marriage. This chapter will help you discern when your body is hungry for food and when your body (mind and heart) is hungry for something besides food. You will be given the opportunity to look at how you use food to cope with your emotions instead of coping with them directly, and what lies underneath this urge to eat. Exploring what you're really hungry for and learning how to skillfully hold your painful emotions without food is where the rubber hits the road on the journey to health and happiness.

This next important step on your journey with food will help you deeply understand your urges to eat when you're bored, restless, sad, happy, and stressed. To aid in the process, this chapter normalizes the unpleasant aspects of our lives. Disappointment, sadness, fear, confusion, and anger are emotions we all feel. But you can learn elegant, simple tools for experiencing your emotions and choosing your responses through a kind, compassionate acknowledgment and exploration of your quite human experience.

A powerful technique for exploring your hunger involves pausing long enough to hear the cry from within for a more authentic life.

Underneath your myriad emotions are messages that lead you to the highest expression of your being. Exploring what you're really hungry for on a regular basis will help you reach for food less often while you engage in creating meaning and happiness in your life. The ultimate goal of mindful eating is to relearn how to eat when you are biologically hungry and how to meet your other needs (emotional, mental, and spiritual) with strategies other than food.

PHYSICAL HUNGER VERSUS CRAVINGS

Teasing apart the difference between sensations of biological hunger due to not having eaten in a while and the bodily response you feel when you are experiencing a craving is complicated by many factors. As we talked about earlier, the sensations associated with biological hunger can feel similar in the body to those you experience when you are distressed. Further, sensations of physical hunger can arise even when there isn't an energy need in the body or prolonged food deprivation. For instance, your body can report hunger when you simply see a plate of cookies or when you walk past a doughnut shop and smell fresh doughnuts being made, even if you've just eaten a full meal (Lowe and Butryn 2007).

Food craving has been described as "a motivational state associated with a strong desire for an expected positive outcome" and "the function of food craving will be to initiate bingeing as a means of obtaining relief from the aversive state of intolerable negative affect" (Waters, Hill, and Waller 2001, 883). In other words, craving food can be driven by a desire to escape from a negative mood or unpleasant emotion, previous attempts at restraining eating, and environmental or social cues. While you might feel temporary relief upon eating at these times, there is a down side. When craving leads to overeating or a binge, your mood is likely to deteriorate even further and, because you're eating more than your body biologically needs, you are likely to gain weight.

However, cravings for food can be differentiated from biological hunger by taking a closer look at what's happening in your body *and* mind. Here are a couple of examples. Kevin was having a stressful day when he drove past a favorite fast food joint and immediately had the thought, *I want some burgers!* Kevin had often used his burger habit to deal with stress, and he recognized this desire as a craving as opposed to biological hunger. Macy was walking downtown when a swarm of cicadas (very big, black, noisy bugs) flew out of a tree and headed straight toward her. Her first thought was *I need a candy bar.* Surprised by the cicadas, she knew she was really just afraid. Kevin and Macy had been practicing mindfulness for a few weeks, so they both had an immediate awareness of how their emotions and thoughts had been triggered by environmental and emotional cues to eat.

By stopping and noticing the stress and the fear, Kevin and Macy had essential learning experiences. They could feel their bodies reacting to stress and fear and hear the thoughts, but not turn to food as a result. In both of these cases, the craving for food left very quickly. Becoming mindfully aware of your bodily reactions, feelings, and thoughts will help you pause instead of react to a craving.

How long does a craving last if you pay attention to it without succumbing to food? I don't have a scientific answer but encourage you to find out for yourself. The next time you experience a craving, see if you can notice what is happening—in your body, feelings, and thoughts. How long does it take a craving to end if you don't act on it? It can't last very long—a few seconds at the least and maybe thirty minutes at the most.

This strategy is similar to one called "urge surfing," designed by Alan Marlatt for people recovering from addictions to cigarettes, alcohol, and other drugs (Marlatt and Kristeller 1999). You can think about your craving, or urge, as a wave in the ocean. Surfing the wave of a craving can teach you how to mindfully be with the sensations until they pass. You can directly observe the changing nature and impermanence of cravings rather than feeding them or fighting with them. You can also redirect your attention to something else and, before you know it, the craving is gone.

In order to be a mindful eater, you will need to understand and befriend your "wanting mind." It says you need more food even though you are full. The wanting mind wants pleasure of any kind it can find—food, clothes, shoes, jewelry, cars, flowers, and so on. Become aware of when you hear the wanting mind grabbing for pleasurable experiences. The important thing to remember is it is insatiable. To the wanting mind, there is never enough. You can become familiar with the wanting mind saying "more" and kindly acknowledge it, but then redirect your attention to the taste and pleasure of the food and the fullness of your body to determine when you stop eating. You can use this same technique with the various emotions you experience that lead to overeating. Befriending your mind and your emotions is the key to changing your relationship to food and your body.

EMOTIONAL EATING

Eating for emotional reasons can become a habit that is hard to break. Food is your BFF (best friend forever). We use eating as a form of relief from boredom, an escape from our feelings, and a substitute for love. It's the quick, easy fix for modern life, which seems altogether too busy to let us stop long enough to ask ourselves what we really need. So, we reach for food instead. Food equals *temporary* happiness and comfort. This strategy works for a hot minute, but then you're left feeling full and probably like a fool (because you didn't meet your actual needs and now you weigh more than you want to). At family gatherings and celebrations involving food, the rules and guilt trips about eating can be particularly problematic and can propel the celebration into a food binge. Let's cover some of the main ways you might use food as something other than nourishment for your body.

Food = Entertainment and Freedom from Boredom

When I ask people why they eat, besides out of physical hunger, many say they eat for entertainment or because they're bored. These are two sides of the same coin. In a world where entertainment is available 24–7, we are constantly bombarded with images, messages, music, and sounds that draw our attention. There is a sense that you need to interact (e.g., Facebook, phone calls, text messaging) or lose yourself in something (e.g., TV show, movie, music, books). Boredom can be described as the absence of stimulation, having nothing to do, not wanting to do anything else, or having things to do but not wanting to do them.

Without something to do or to distract you when you are bored, you are left with yourself to contend with. This is when things can get challenging. The lack of stimulation can feel uncomfortable and unsettling if you aren't used to it. In the emptiness, emotions such as loneliness, sadness, restlessness, or worry begin to surface that have not had the space to be heard. Feelings of guilt can arise because of the belief that you "should" be doing something to be productive. And, when you feel uneasy, food is an easy, fast, cheap way to fill the void. Eating food becomes something to "do" so uncomfortable emotions don't have to be experienced.

The moments of having nothing encroaching on your senses but the natural world around you are precious few, unless you purposely set aside time for them. And, for many people, spending time in silence—"being" instead of "doing"—is not prioritized or cultivated. Now is the perfect time to practice your mindfulness. Be curious about why the lack of activity, stimulation, or entertainment is experienced as uncomfortable. Become curious about this thing called "boredom" until you understand experientially what is going on underneath the word. Bringing mindful attention to anything, even boredom, makes it inherently more interesting. In fact, boredom and mindfulness are psychologically incompatible states.

When you explore boredom, you have the opportunity to just sit and feel whatever emotions might be present with kindness and compassion. You might also uncover an interest in something that would bring you pleasure and engage in it. Halley said, "I've noticed that when I'm bored, what I usually want is to be creative. I love creating— whether it's drawing, crafting, painting, or jewelry making. I'm a creative nut. I discovered a couple of weeks ago I love making bread. Just the act of stirring up the ingredients, kneading the dough and shaping it is something that gives me enormous amounts of pleasure. When I was holding the ball of dough, I realized I was smiling like a Cheshire cat! Of course, it was delicious when baked, too. Bonus!"

Discover what it is you want to do that makes you happy or find out what it's like to sit with yourself without needing to do anything. Relearning to delight in being with yourself, befriending yourself, is one of the greatest gifts you can give and receive.

Food = Comfort and Escape

You've had a bad day at work, the kids have gotten on your nerves, your friend stood you up for lunch, your spouse pissed you off at breakfast, or maybe you just had a bad commute home. Something to eat and drink sounds just like the ticket to feeling better. It is quite common to use food and drink as a way of cheering yourself up or escaping from the things you'd rather forget. Food tastes delicious and alcohol numbs the pain. For a brief time you have a pleasurable experience, instead of feeling frustrated and stressed. Your mood turns around—momentarily.

While on rare occasion this scenario is not necessarily destructive, it is easy to see how if you eat (or drink) for comfort or escape on a regular basis, this becomes problematic. Although food can be delicious and give you pleasure, it isn't designed to make you feel happy. It's designed to give you energy to live. If you are using food as your coping mechanism for stress, you will end up weighing more than you want. Gaining weight will lead to feelings of guilt and frustration, which takes you back to food again. You can run to the kitchen to escape the world, but you can't hide the weight that you put on during the trip.

Food = Love

Looking for love (or any of our other needs) in all the wrong places is so common that it's the title of a famous country music song. Judy, a nurse who works in a hospital, said it is very difficult to eat healthily where she works. She is constantly on the go and doesn't have time to care for herself by eating lunch, drinking water, or even making it to the bathroom. "I only have time to take care of my patients. Chocolate equals love," she said, "and that's what I go for in the middle of my busy day."

We feed ourselves and we feed others in order to show our love. We don't mean to harm. However, when giving food becomes the way to show our love and eating is the way to return that love, we suffer not only from weight gain but from lack of true intimacy and connection. Learning how to express love to yourself and others in ways besides food may take a little extra time and even be a little scary, but it could save you from the misery of overeating and will ultimately enhance your relationships.

When you substitute food for entertainment, comfort, or love, you have fallen into a habit that pacifies you temporarily. Like any habit, you keep doing it because it provides you with at least occasional moments of enjoyment. Until now you might not have had any better strategies to employ.

What follows is a profound teaching that can free you from emotional eating and more. The only way to navigate your path to freedom is right through the middle of your unpleasant emotions and circumstances. You cannot pass "Go." You cannot take a detour. Your reward for bravely and compassionately facing the unpleasant aspects of your life will be your ability to handle anything life brings your way with grace and equanimity. It is truly worth the trip.

UNDERSTANDING AND ACCEPTING UNPLEASANT EMOTIONS

If you are anything like most people, you didn't have a class in "how to deal with difficult emotions" when you were in grade school, a time in which such a thing could have been really useful. If you had, it might have kept you from developing less-than-helpful habits such as eating, drinking, shopping, fighting, blaming, and other destructive tendencies designed to avoid and deny your feelings. Fred Rogers, the late host of *Mister Rogers' Neighborhood*, said, "If we can teach children that feelings are mentionable and manageable, we will have done a great service for mental health" (Ryan 2013, 83). Even if you didn't learn healthy ways of dealing with your feelings when you were young, it is never too late to bring compassion and understanding to your world of emotions. It is never too late to realize that all emotions are *mentionable* and *manageable*, and I'd like to add *natural*.

First of all, unpleasant emotions are natural and mentionable. Everyone has them and will continue to have them as long as they are alive. They are a part of us and arise out of the conditions of our existence. Even the most enlightened human beings you know have feelings of sadness and anger. They, like you, feel deeply from the heart. Unpleasant emotions are not bad or wrong. They are a natural and normal part of our shared human existence.

It's helpful to understand that for at least half of your life you will feel a little to a lot of physical or emotional discomfort. It is not your birthright to have only pleasant experiences, so maintaining that position is only going to set you up to feel even worse. When you insist you should only be happy, you will have the pain of the difficult emotion and the pain of your resistance to it. Your ability to be with the unpleasant without having to fix, deny, avoid, or run away is crucial to your physical, emotional, mental, and spiritual well-being. The only way to fully experience the joy in your life is to go through the work of feeling the pain.

The first step is awareness. What are you feeling? Since you might not be used to doing this, I suggest you check in with yourself throughout the day. Name and acknowledge what feeling is present—happiness, frustration, confusion, and so on. Putting your feelings into words, called "affect labeling," can help you regulate a negative experience by changing a part of your brain associated with emotions and subsequent reactions (Lieberman et al. 2007). In other words, knowing what you're feeling can give you a little distance from it, allowing you to take a deep breath (literally and metaphorically).

Once you have identified what you're feeling (and taken a deep breath), you are on your way to managing it. You don't have to like it or want it, but accepting that a feeling is present (because it is) is a sane approach to reality. You will never win a fight with a difficult emotion. "Whatever you fight, you strengthen, and what you resist, persists" (Tolle 2005, 75). If you face an emotion, acknowledge it, label it, and accept its presence, then it will begin to soften and eventually fade away. All emotions (just like everything else in life) are impermanent and manageable.

MANAGING YOUR EMOTIONS

After you initially acknowledge and accept that an emotion is present, there are more and less skillful approaches to take next.

Letting emotions run wild, like unruly children, might temporarily relieve some built-up tension. However, the more you give them free rein, the more likely they are to proliferate and magnify. Whatever you practice, you get better at. If you practice being angry or impatient, you will get better at being angry or impatient. On the other hand, repressing emotions is also an unhelpful strategy and has been associated with serious mental and physical problems.

Although it can often feel like you are at the mercy of your emotions, there are a number of ways of managing them so they aren't managing you. The key is to feel your emotions (without repressing them) while working to transform your relationship to them. The three main methods for partnering with your emotions are *mindfulness of emotions, broadening the focus,* and *learning the lesson.* The first method is essential for understanding how to be with emotions without feeling overwhelmed, the second allows you to experience the full spectrum of your emotions instead of getting stuck on just one, and the third helps you use your emotions to understand and navigate the circumstances involved.

Mindfulness of Emotions

The ability to be mindful of your emotions requires a willingness to be awake and aware of your humanity from moment to moment. Instead of numbing out with food or denying your emotions, it takes great courage to feel your emotions directly. Even with all of the kindness and compassion you can muster, a difficult emotion will still feel uncomfortable. While some pain is inevitable, the need to suffer or eat away the pain is optional. Mindfulness teaches you that you will not only survive the difficult emotion, but you will thrive as a result of having met it fully.

Let's go into the process of mindfully attending to your emotions in more detail, step by step. So, take a deep breath and let's get started.

1. *Acknowledge the emotion that is currently present.* The first step is to know what you're feeling. This is harder than it sounds. When you first feel an emotion, name it as best you can (it may morph into something else as you examine it more closely). Let's use sadness as an example. Instead of saying *I'm sad*, try something like *I'm aware of sadness* or simply *Sadness is present*. Taking the "I" out of the statement begins to take the personal out of the emotion. You might also try *Sadness is just what wants to be here right now*. This approach acknowledges the impermanent nature of emotions. It begins to help you understand that you and "sadness" are not synonymous and to experience sadness as a passing phenomenon.

2. *Notice what the emotion feels like in the body.* Where do you feel a particular emotion in your body? It might be tightness in your chest, a pain in your stomach, or a clenched jaw. Whatever it is, just notice with curiosity and kindness. Notice whether it changes under your examination and how. Difficult emotions are actually triggered by a bodily reaction to something in your internal or external environment that is determined to be a threat. Take your time to discover what an emotion feels like in your body.

3. *Notice what thoughts are present.* Thoughts and feelings go hand in hand. Once your body registers something as threatening and sends a signal to the emotional center of your brain (the limbic system), a half a second later a message reaches the thinking brain (the neocortex) and you have a thought. Generally the first thoughts will be some kind of cognitive distortion in reaction to the emotions and bodily sensations. Your thinking will be shaded by the emotion, but as we learned in the last chapter, thoughts

aren't facts. Simply see the thought as a thought and let it go instead of running it over and over in your head.

4. *Actively move toward the emotion.* Once you are aware of what you are feeling, what sensations are present in your body, and what thoughts are present, you have dropped out of automatic pilot and are fully awake to the present. Now the important work becomes staying with your current emotional experience. This is often a time when you will want to run away, fight, and resist—or eat—or do anything except stay present. Instead of these old strategies, *do nothing.* When a difficult feeling such as sadness arises, tell yourself with kindness, *Sadness is present. This is just what wants to be here right now.* I have found this practice to be amazingly helpful. At this point, you might discover another related emotion. Acknowledge and sit beside any emotion that arises.

5. *Keep coming back to the feeling.* You might find yourself going back to the thoughts that feed the feeling. This could be a thought about another person, about yourself, about your life. The subject doesn't matter. Extract your attention from the subject to the direct experience of the emotion. Without a subject to spark the emotion, the emotion becomes fluid; it cannot sustain itself for very long. It's like a fire. If you don't keep putting sticks on the fire, the fire will eventually extinguish. If you don't keep feeding an emotion with your thoughts, the emotion will soon run out of flames.

Broadening the Focus

This method for working with your emotions is intended to help you break out of the trance of a particular emotion. Sometimes you can get so focused on being irritated with someone that you forget the other people you find quite pleasant. Or, you might be so obsessed with thinking about food, you have a hard time engaging with the rest of the world around you. It's like you're using a zoom lens on your camera instead of the landscape lens. Broadening the focus is about remembering to take in the landscape of your life.

Here are some examples. If you are mad at someone, you can continue to feed the irritation or you can shift gears. Think about all of the people in your life you aren't mad at. Bring those people to mind and think about the loving parts of your relationships with them. In addition, there may be wonderful aspects of your relationship with the person you are mad at. Bring your kinder memories to mind and notice the associated emotions. Anger has a hard time coexisting with love. You will be feeling one or the other. Cultivating love is a way of neutralizing the anger. Spending time consciously nurturing positive emotions will leave less time for the difficult emotions to overcome you.

When people are first learning to stop eating before they are stuffed, they sometimes experience anxiety. That place of "not hungry, not full" can feel empty and scary at first. While your belly may feel anxious, practice shifting your attention to another part of your body—a part that feels neutral and safe—and focus your attention there. When your attention moves back to the anxiety in your belly, with great kindness move your attention to the safe part of your body.

Have you gotten into a habit of thinking about food and feeling overwhelmed by it? If this is happening, practice bringing your attention to what is actually happening in the present moment. Engage with the work in front of you or the people around you. You can choose to do something as simple as taking a walk and mindfully experiencing your body moving. You can engage in an activity, such as cleaning out a closet, playing the piano, or calling a friend. Anything you can do to break the trance of the emotionally charged situation will be beneficial.

By broadening (or shifting) the focus from a difficult emotion to a neutral, safe, or enjoyable emotion, you are training the mind that you are in control. You are managing the difficult emotions and cultivating the positive and pleasant. The intention of this practice is not for you to repress or run away from an emotion, but to help you determine the times when you need to take action to improve your well-being.

Happiness is a choice, and you are learning to see that there are many things we can choose to focus on at any moment. The more you focus on the uplifting and nurturing, the more joy you will experience in your life. When you are consumed with worry, anger, or sadness, take a deep breath and ask yourself, *In this moment, where is my freedom from suffering?* Notice both the answer and any resistance to the answer. It can be difficult to break out of our habits of suffering. Let your mindfulness practice help you cultivate the joy.

Learning the Lesson

This next method is about fully appreciating and responding skillfully to any important information that may be conveyed by an emotion. For instance, if you get angry after someone yells at you, pay attention to what the anger is telling you. First, it is saying *I don't like being talked to like that.* It is also giving you information about the person who is yelling. The person could have had a really bad day and is unwittingly taking it out on you. Or, the person might have a pattern of yelling at you. The anger can be a catalyst for you to do something in response—set appropriate boundaries, have a conversation (after the person has calmed down) about how being yelled at makes you feel, or inquire into what is troubling this person.

Emotions can help mobilize us to action in order to create environments that are nurturing, healing, and enriching. The dark nights (or moments) of our soul are highly underrated. It is often because of difficult times that we gain clarity, insight, humor, and inspiration.

Particularly when you have the same emotion over and over again, this is an ideal time to pay attention to the lesson it holds for you. There is no need to make someone else accountable for your emotion and there is no "wrong" emotion. Accepting the lesson of your emotions and managing them skillfully will greatly decrease the need to run to food when a difficulty arises.

WHAT ARE YOU REALLY, REALLY, REALLY HUNGRY FOR?

Eating will only satisfy your physical hunger. If you're eating to satisfy emotional, mental, or spiritual hunger, you might have moments when these needs go underground, but you will never feel satisfied. The only way to end emotional eating is to start looking directly at all of your needs, values, desires, and dreams and decide how you will meet them. You will eat when you're hungry, breathe when you're stressed, laugh when you're happy, play when you're bored, move when your body needs to stretch, learn when your mind needs to expand, and love when your heart aches to be broken open.

So when you find yourself reaching for food but you suspect it may not be because you're physically hungry, ask yourself, *What am I hungry for?* The first answer might be a chocolate brownie.

Ask again, *What am I really, really hungry for?* Take a moment to pause and look a little deeper. Are you physically hungry? Are you wanting a bite of a chocolate brownie because you think it would be lovely to savor one right now? Or do you notice anxiety, fear, confusion, sadness, loneliness, grief, anger, exhaustion, or tension? If distressing feelings aren't present, you might go ahead and mindfully have your chocolate brownie.

However, if you notice emotional discomfort of some kind, ask yourself again, *What am I really, really, really hungry for?* In other words, *What do I need right now that would address the feelings I'm experiencing or meet my underlying needs?* The answer to this question won't be found in the bottom of the cookie jar, a bag of chips, or a chocolate brownie.

Discovering how to meet your difficult emotions by sitting mindfully with them or by responding with some kind of skillful action will take investigation, trial and error, courage, and honesty. You can work at this on a couple of different levels. First, you can address and honor your immediate needs, and second, you can work on discovering (or rediscovering) your values and dreams. The first step will prepare you to take the second step and delve into the deeper examination of your life that I braced you for at the beginning of the book.

Honoring Your Immediate Needs

Immediate needs usually fall into the category of physiological needs. When you ask yourself the question "What am I really, really, *really* hungry for?" your immediate need might be as simple as attending to the body by moving, stretching, or lying down for a short nap. Sleep is a highly overlooked need, the lack of which is causing people lots of physical and psychological discomfort. You might need a break from the computer or TV—even if it's a thirty-second break to take some deep breaths while you're in the bathroom. You might need to go outside and breathe some fresh air or take in the smells and sights of nature. You might need to drink some water. Hydration is often what people are really needing when they reach for food. While these all sound simple, our basic physical needs often get overlooked in our too-busy-to-stop culture.

Discovering Your Values and Dreams

Once you've met your immediate needs, it's time to take a deeper dive. If you haven't been paying attention, life might be dragging you along for a ride you didn't intend to take. Looking at where you are now and where you want to be will be an essential step in designing the architecture of your life as well as ending the habit of emotional eating. This step requires your full participation and full responsibility. While you can gather support along the way, no one else has your answers and no one else can do the heavy lifting. When you're busy creating your most meaningful life, food and eating may be a part of that scenario, but they aren't the fix for what you've neglected to take care of.

So what *are* you really, really, really hungry for? Do you know? This question can only be answered in the present. You might have known at some time in the past, but if you haven't checked in for a while, that answer might have changed. How alive is your answer and how does the answer feel in your gut? This is a question you can ask yourself over and over again. Dive every day into your heart and listen to what it tells you. This can be a great time to pull out your journal and give your pen free rein over the page.

Your needs can be quite varied and can be fulfilled in countless ways. Your emotional needs in relationships can be for acceptance, acknowledgment, appreciation, and attention and can be met by asking for what you want and setting appropriate boundaries. Needs for creativity can be met in infinite ways—cooking, writing, painting, home decorating, golfing, gardening, singing, playing a musical instrument, and even in projects we do at work. Career needs tend to relate to expressing our personal selves in the work that we do and can be met by defining our values and figuring out how to articulate them on the job. Mental needs can be fulfilled by engagement of our brain in figuring out problems, learning new information and skills, and exploring the world from top to bottom. Spiritual needs can be met by being in nature, engaging in a church or spiritual community, and listening to inspiring talks or reading inspiring books.

To get back in harmony with your deeper needs and hungers, taking an inventory of your values and evaluating the degree to which you are living them can be enlightening. Living in harmony with your values is one of the most supportive ways to meet your physical, emotional, mental, and spiritual needs. For instance, one of my values is health. Since health is a value I deeply hold, I make exercise and eating green vegetables non-negotiable priorities. I don't even have to think about it anymore. I just do it, because I have made a clear, conscious decision that health is important to me.

Fear can be a very limiting emotion when it comes to our dreams and aspirations. Fear disconnects us from our heart and our inner wisdom. It disconnects us from what really matters. Ask yourself, *What would I do if I weren't afraid?* Give yourself time to explore the variety of answers that arise in response to this question. You don't necessarily have to jump from a plane, leave your husband, or quit your job, but you might at some point. Start with some smaller things you are afraid of and work your way up. Imagine yourself doing the things you would be afraid to do and then do them. There is power in your mind that you barely access. When we do those things that we fear, we develop self-confidence and resilience. Following your yearnings will be energizing and motivating.

Psychologist Steven Hayes was quoted as saying, "The natural game most of us are in is how to *feel* good. That's not the same thing as how to *live* good" (Traister 2006). Living good is about discovering your deepest values, setting intentions for yourself that honor them, and taking action on them. Take some time with your journal to help clarify your values and provide vision for your life. Use some of the strategies and questions that I've posed to help guide your reflections.

I know I've given you a lot to think about, but please don't let that scare you away. Your hungers in life cannot all be met in one day, one week, or even one year. The key is to write down some specific goals (or even one goal) and move toward them regularly. If you don't know where you want to go, you won't know what steps to take to get there. Once you have set an intention, there is power and magic to it. Every small step that you take is huge compared to taking no step at all. In fact, focusing on the small steps is so much easier and less overwhelming. Every big dream comprises thousands of small steps. Take one today.

EMOTIONALLY RENEWING YOURSELF

Taking preventative measures on a regular basis to boost your emotional bank account can help reduce the amount of time you feel emotionally bankrupt. If your emotional bank account is flush, you will be much less likely to turn to food as a fix. This does not have to take a long time every day or every week, but it does need to be consistent. Your emotional energy can be enhanced by engaging in any activity that is pleasurable and uplifting (Loehr and Schwartz 2003). These pleasurable activities inoculate you against stress and other challenges of life.

Julia Cameron (2002), in her wonderful book on creativity called *The Artist's Way*, asks readers to engage in a weekly "artist's date." This is a time to set aside for yourself, at least once a week, to do something just for you—something you would find engaging, fun, and pleasurable. Since many people don't set aside time for themselves, this can be a bit of a challenge. Don't fall prey to the tendency of doing everything for everyone else and leaving yourself out in the cold. You are the most important person in your life. Now is the time to start acting like it!

Exercise: Forgiveness Practice

In the process of letting go of emotional eating, it will be helpful to let go of the judgments you have harbored against yourself and others. They are both equally harmful, and as long as they eat at you, you will be vulnerable to overeating and the self-loathing from which it comes. The regrets about the ways you haven't honored your deepest needs might have turned into shame and guilt, which need the soft embrace of a forgiving heart.

From a mindfulness perspective, you have no need to be forgiven, but this must be comprehended at an experiential level. Forgiveness practice can guide you to a cellular understanding that all can be released and all is well in this moment. Grieving and letting go of the past is an essential part of moving forward, of truly knowing you don't need to *be* any different than you are, *do* anything to be better, or *look* any different.

Forgiveness is not something that can be forced, and you don't have to feel a particular way when you do this exercise. Let the power of your intention and your willingness to even try it at all be enough to start. You can download an audio recording of this exercise at http://newharbinger.com/33278 or http://www.lynnrossy.com.

Start by finding a comfortable sitting position and bring your attention to your body as a whole and the breath within the body. Be aware of the sensations in your body from head to toe to fingertip. As you scan the body, imagine tension leaving with each out-breath and light and energy coming in with each in-breath. Let your mind and body relax.

After a moment or two of settling into your body and your breath, let your attention move to your heart center. Breathe in and out gently from the center of your chest—your heart center. Feel the energy of your beating, human heart. Take your time. There is no need to hurry. When your mind wanders, keep coming to the breath at the center of your chest.

Feel how precious it is to be alive and breathing in this moment. Feel how precious you are at your very core. And, offer yourself these words. Breathe them into your heart and let them infuse your body with forgiveness.

I forgive myself for all of the ways that I have been less than loving toward myself. *Then let your past unkind and destructive thoughts and actions come into your awareness and release them one by one. On the other side of the coin, let the things you wish you would have said and done, but didn't, come into your awareness and release them one by one. Tell yourself,* I am so sorry for the hurt and pain that I have caused. And, in this moment, I accept, love, and forgive myself.

It might feel good to place your hands over your heart center. Feel the warmth and softness of your human body. Feel the beating of your human heart. Feel your common humanity with all people who seek understanding and forgiveness.

*Breathe, relax, and prepare yourself for the next phrase—*I forgive others for all of the ways they have been less than loving toward me. *Then let the people whom you have not forgiven come to mind. You do not have to condone the words they said or the actions they took which have been painful and hurtful to you. But, as each person or circumstance comes to mind, say to him or her,* I release you, your words, and your actions that have hurt me. I know that if I hold on to this hurt, I will only be hurting myself. In the service of my healing and well-being, I forgive you.

Take another moment to gently breath in and out through the center of your chest—the heart center. Feel the heart from which all love and forgiveness arise. Let your mind and body relax. Breathe out any tension and breathe in light and energy into the heart and the rest of your body.

*Breathe, relax, and prepare yourself for the next phrase—*I forgive myself for all of the ways I have been less than loving toward others. *Let the past unkind and destructive thoughts and actions you have directed toward others come into your awareness. As each person comes to mind whom you may have* *harmed, imagine there is a stream of light connecting his or her heart and yours. Tell each person,* I am so sorry for the hurt and pain that I may have caused you. And, in this moment, I ask for your forgiveness.

Take a few more moments to sit quietly with yourself, your breath, and your beating heart. Many different emotions may arise. Let them wash through the openness of your heart center. Breathe with them and let them move, shift, and flow naturally. And, when you are ready, opening your eyes and taking in the sights of the room.

Forgiveness is something that happens not just once, but over time. Peeling off the layers of emotions that may have hardened over the years requires patience and trust. Give them time to soften and release. Make forgiveness a part of your regular meditation or reflections for the day.

CHALLENGES:

- The habit of emotional eating has a temporary payoff, and food is fast and easy.

- The entertainment culture creates an environment where it's easy to become disconnected from your body, mind, and heart.

- Facing difficult emotions directly instead of eating to drown them out can be uncomfortable and requires courage and compassion.

- Digging deep and knowing what you're really, really, really hungry for takes time and exploration.

- Forgiving yourself and others takes practice and won't happen in one sitting.

THE GOOD NEWS

- Emotions are natural and normal, mentionable and manageable.

- Mindfulness teaches you how to be with emotions without running away from them or stuffing them with food.

- There are always positives in your life to focus on, no matter how bad things are. All you have to do is broaden your focus to include them in your awareness.

- You know what you want and need, but you might have forgotten to ask. The answers are just waiting to be heard.

- Forgiveness is a gift you give yourself; it can free you from the past and leave you open to the future.

WHAT YOU CAN DO NOW:

- Mindfulness of Emotions: Keep track of how you are feeling throughout the day. Remember to take the "I" out of the statement and use a phrase such as *Sadness is present*. Don't try to fix it, but acknowledge and breathe with the emotions that pass through your awareness. This practice will help you see the impermanent nature of emotions and teach you they are mentionable and manageable. Ride the wave!

- Do something pleasurable and enjoyable as often as possible to renew your emotional bank account.

- Forgiveness Practice: This exercise will help you uncover where you have been holding anger, shame, guilt, or resentment. You may need to repeat this several times before you get a sense of release. Keep your forgiveness practice alive by including it in a daily reflection or by journaling. At the end of the day, review how you have treated yourself and others and how you have felt treated by them. As each thought or action occurs to you, if needed, send forgiveness to yourself and others.

CHAPTER 7

Moving in Ways That
Feel Delicious

In order to savor delicious food, you have to pay attention to how it tastes. In order to move in ways that feel delicious, you have to bring your full attention to your bodily sensations. Whether you currently enjoy exercising or not, mindfulness can make the experience of moving your body a pleasurable one, teach you to embrace the instrumental value of the body, protect you from injury, and help you make appropriate adjustments to how you move as you grow older.

You may have some resistance to paying attention to your body, particularly if you and your body aren't exactly on friendly terms. You may be unhappy with your body for the way it looks, for the way it feels, or for not living up to your expectations. You also might think you're too busy to pay attention to the body and its needs for movement or may find the idea of exercise unappealing. As a result, like many people, you may have neglected your body's need to be active.

This chapter will help you use mindfulness of your body as a way of deeply and gently listening to what it needs and wants in terms of movement and activity. Bringing kind attention to your body throughout the day can illuminate when it wants a break, a stretch, a walk, or to breathe more deeply. As you will read, you don't need a gym membership, special clothes, or a lot of time to feel, move, stretch, and strengthen your body in ways that feel delicious. Finding your favorite way to become physically active can happen when you are willing to explore your body with an open, curious attitude.

Research presented in this chapter demonstrates the importance of engaging in movement throughout the day to improve your well-being. By taking small steps to be more active, the body can respond in amazing ways such as with improved blood pressure, decreased body fat and weight, and help regulating the way you eat.

THE EXERCISE DILEMMA

Are you a person who can't wait to exercise, or would you rather not think about it? For some, just the word "exercise" is a turn off. Exercise may conjure up visions of the gym, being miserable doing some activity you don't like to do, being around people who make you feel self-conscious (muscle-bound men and women in tight spandex), or being in pain. That doesn't sound too enticing, does it?

Further, while exercise is very beneficial, it can become a drudgery because of its association with weight loss and dieting. You might tell yourself you have to exercise as a way of balancing out any extra morsel of food you put into your mouth, while the enjoyment of movement is completely overlooked or squashed. Using exercise exclusively for weight loss takes the pleasure out of the activity because the focus is on something other than how it makes you feel inside.

Other common reasons for not exercising are the lack of time, insufficient energy, and not knowing what to do. There is the belief that you must work out for at least an hour before it counts, sweat a lot, and shower before you do anything else. If you are uncomfortable with your weight or how your body looks, you might think you need a better body before you even get started. Jonie, a mother of two young children, used to ride her bike regularly before her children were born. After seeing her weight steadily rise over the past few years, she said, "I don't want anyone to see the fat person exercising." She needed some help rediscovering the joy of movement.

Overcoming resistance to exercise can be as simple as redefining what it means to you and deciding not to listen to the voices in your head that tell you to stay on the couch. As I mentioned in an earlier chapter, thoughts aren't facts, and that applies to the negative thoughts you have about exercising. When Nancy started exploring her resistance to exercise, she said, "In the time I spend arguing with myself about exercise, I could have completed an hour workout." If your mind is full of reasons why you shouldn't move your body, just mindfully acknowledge them. There are plenty of tips in this chapter to help you get moving in spite of them.

ORNAMENTAL VERSUS INSTRUMENTAL VIEW OF THE BODY

In western society, most girls are acculturated to view their body as an object, with a focus on its shape or attractiveness, and judge themselves accordingly—an "ornamental" view. Boys, on the other hand, are generally acculturated to view their body in terms of its function and how well it performs—an "instrumental" view. While girls have suffered from the inability to live up to extremely harsh body standards, boys have suffered from the inability to be strong enough or competitive enough in sports. However, research indicates that when you shift your focus to how the body functions (an instrumental view) rather than its form (an ornamental view) you have a more positive evaluation of your body (Gusella, Clark, and van Roosmalen 2004).

Do you ever stop and thank your body for the incredible feats it does every day? Your eyes can see, your tongue can taste, your ears can hear, and your nose can smell. Your body can digest food, eliminate toxins, pump blood through your heart, protect itself from disease, and take in vital oxygen. Your legs and feet take you where you want to go and your arms and hands carry things for you, feed you, and hug your loved ones.

Take a moment right now and thank your body for three wonderful functions it performs. Do this every day and see if you notice a deeper kinship with your body. When you feel better about your body, you are more likely to take care of its needs and take it out for some regular activity.

EVERY MOVEMENT COUNTS

James Levine, who conducts research at the Mayo Clinic, suggests we should all stand up, move around more, and even fidget as a way of preventing many chronic diseases produced by a sedentary lifestyle. He coined the term non-exercise activity thermogenesis (NEAT), which is the energy expenditure of everything we do that is not sleeping, eating, or sports-like exercise (Levine et al. 2006). Interestingly, NEAT accounts for most of our energy expenditure in the day, over and above exercise. And, if we increase the time we spend in NEAT activity, we could improve overall health as well as reduce the risk of metabolic syndrome, cardiovascular events, and "all-cause" mortality (Villablanca et al. 2015).

You do not have to do an hour of intense activity every day. The most important thing is to move your body whenever possible. When you know that every movement counts, you might be more eager to do household chores, rake the leaves, walk to the store, do exercises while you're watching TV, park farther away from work or the store, or put on music and dance while you clean. When you notice how good it feels to move your body, you might surprise yourself at how much more you can move during the day.

Joyce was so obese she could barely walk, much less exercise. Yet she was so determined, she started spending extra time pushing her shopping cart (using it like a walker for support). After a while, when it got easier, she added bags of dog food—first, small ones, then multiple large bags, to the point where customers repeatedly asked her if it was on sale! She went on to tolerating more strenuous activity, became healthy, and lost a bunch of weight. I love that story! It demonstrates that anybody can find a way to pick up the pace (or add a few laps around the grocery store!).

MAKE YOUR WORKPLACE ACTIVE

Workplaces are so sedentary that sitting has become the new smoking. In a study of 123,216 people followed over a fourteen-year period, women who spent six hours or more a day sitting had a 37 percent increased risk of dying compared to those who spent less than three hours a day sitting, regardless of their physical activity level during the rest of the day (Patel et al. 2010). This means that even exercising at night for an hour will not overcome the negative effects on the body of sitting for long periods of time.

To get more NEAT activity at work, think about how you can restructure your day. Give your body a break every sixty to ninety minutes throughout the day to walk or stretch, take the stairs instead of the elevator, use the bathroom on a different floor, implement walking meetings, stand at meetings and when you're on the phone, use an exercise ball at your desk, use a sit-stand desk, and walk to talk to a coworker instead of sending an email. Not only will you feel better, but engaging in physical activity may suppress the drive to overeat caused by cognitive stress that builds up at work (Joseph et al. 2010).

I often encounter people who believe that changing the work culture is prohibitive—mainly due to being stuck in the old way of doing things and the fear of change. But, with a little imagination and courage, you can be the ambassador for health for you and your coworkers. Microbreaks (as they are called in the ergonomic literature) can be from thirty seconds to five minutes and many can even be done at your desk. Break out of your rut at work and shake it up a little!

THE BENEFITS OF PAYING ATTENTION

An interesting study by Ellen Langer demonstrated something pretty startling about the body and the benefits of paying attention. Langer surveyed hotel maids and discovered that 67 percent of those questioned didn't see themselves as physically active—which seems a little bizarre considering the amount of work they do all day. She took two groups of maids and measured their body fat, waist-to-hip ratio, blood pressure, weight, and body mass index. One group was informed that the activity they engaged in during their work day defined them as having an "active lifestyle" according to the Centers for Disease Control and Prevention. The other group was given no information at all. One month later, the physical measurements were taken again, and the women who had been educated demonstrated a decrease in blood pressure, weight, and waist-to-hip ratio while the other group did not (Crum and Langer 2007). The implication is that if you are aware you are exercising and believe you are exercising, your body may respond more than if you are not aware. The placebo effect should not to be underrated, but used to your advantage.

In addition, a study of 398 Dutch participants indicates that the more mindful you are when you engage in physical activity, the more satisfaction you will experience (Tsafou et al. 2015). These results were particularly true for people who had a weak habit of physical activity (as measured by the Self-Report Habit Index). And, when you start to notice how good it feels, it can produce some surprising changes. One couple that I counseled used to argue about who *has to* walk the dog, and now they argue about who *gets to* walk the dog!

MOVING AS YOU AGE OR ARE INJURED

We are all prone to injury, and no one can escape aging. As the effects of injury or aging visit you, instead of focusing on what you can't do anymore (and making yourself miserable as a result), it is quite important to generate appreciation for what you *can* do. Especially if you are someone who has been quite active but can no longer participate in a treasured physical pastime, it helps to keep a positive focus. This attitude is hard to maintain in a culture that glorifies strength and competition and lacks empathy for or understanding of the aging process.

Instead of "No Pain, No Gain," remember my motto, "No Pain, No Pain." If you start slowly with any kind of activity, then you are less likely to hurt yourself and you can enjoy the activity in a safe environment. If you mindfully pay attention to your body and respect the messages it sends you, you will be able to nurture the body with patience and kindness, even when your body needs to adjust to circumstances beyond your control. For instance, you can let go of the idea that you should be able to run five miles because you could when you were eighteen years old.

Judy, a sixty-nine-year-old retired school teacher, said, "I might not be able to do the latest Zumba or Jazzercise class, but I love to walk, bike, garden, and do yoga. I treasure every time my body responds with strength and ease. Knowing that every year my options for movement and activity might become less and less makes me very determined to make movement a number one option for my daily life." What wise advice for all of us!

LET'S GET STARTED

The four most important things you can do to make physical activity an enjoyable part of your life are find something you truly like doing, be consistent, schedule it into your day, and visualize yourself as someone who is physically active. It can also be helpful to start with small, realistic goals. This will help you get the most pleasure from the experience without injuring yourself.

Make It Enjoyable

Take your time and explore different kinds of activity until you find what you really enjoy. Remember that a little bit of activity scattered throughout your day is as good as a long workout at the end of the day. Here are just a few examples of the hundreds of things you could do: hike in nature, rock climb, take dance lessons, play with your kids, do Tai Chi or qigong, take a yoga class, try adult gymnastics, use the Wii, ride your bike on a trail, join a club or league, play golf, go for a swim, paddle a kayak or canoe, go skating (or join a derby team), play soccer, join a softball team, play volleyball, go skiing, go scuba diving, go bowling, or simply take a walk.

Remember to ease into any new activity, even it if is as simple as walking. Gradually increase the time you do something so the body can begin to strengthen and accommodate the new demands on it. Stretching is always good but is especially important before and after you engage in strenuous activity. And, learn the proper form for any new activity you engage in so that you reduce the risk of injury. Even walking or biking can be done in a way that injures you. Do a little research before you start and you might prevent a challenging setback.

Be Consistent

Physical activity is a contributing factor to health and well-being as you age, and the negative consequences from not engaging in it can be reversed at any time in your life. The more consistent you are about moving your body, the more benefits you will receive. Being consistent not only supports your physical health but also helps you turn an activity into a routine. There are many theories about how many days it takes to form a habit. My own personal view is you should try something regularly for at least a month to see if you want to make it a part of your routine.

Schedule Activity into Your Day

Probably the best way to be consistent is to schedule it into your day. I worked with Gloria, who insisted she didn't have time to exercise. After brainstorming with her for quite some time, she agreed to walk ten minutes after work before she engaged with her family in the evening. By the end of ten weeks, not only had she accomplished this goal, but she was walking the dog twice a day and walking with her daughter as a way of connecting with her. She said that learning she could fit physical activity into her day was the most important thing she gained from the program.

Visualize Yourself as an Active Person

There will be days when you won't feel like getting your shoes on and going out for a walk or whatever activity you regularly choose to do. But, if you have the vision of yourself as someone who is physically active, something almost magical happens. You don't have to feel like doing it before you start out, you don't have to wait to hear *Oh boy, I get to go take a walk*. On those days when your mind says *I don't feel like it*, the knowledge that you view yourself as someone who values exercise kicks in and you do it anyway.

Imagery has been used successfully to help people do everything from overcoming anxiety to performing well at sports. When you imagine yourself doing something in the future, you can see and feel yourself doing it with complete confidence and great joy. Imagine yourself moving in ways that feel delicious and your body performing at its very peak.

Envisioning your active self is step one in becoming an intrinsic exerciser (Kimiecik 2009). The intrinsic exerciser is motivated to be active because it feels good, not to reach a goal or look better. Valuing the intrinsic aspects of exercise versus the extrinsic aspects has been shown to positively predict physical self-worth, self-reported exercise behavior, and psychological well-being, as well as reduce anxiety about exercising (Sebire, Standage, and Vansteenkiste 2009).

Make Your Plan

What's one enjoyable activity that you can commit to doing consistently and schedule into your day? Can you picture yourself doing it and feeling great? Watch out for when your mind tries to reject the idea that you could be joyously physically active. You may be dealing with some old patterns and conditioning that are limiting you. Listen to your body for the messages it gives you and feel the satisfaction and benefits of becoming embodied. Your new habit of moving will soon take hold and you will hardly even think about taking some extra steps—it will just happen.

Karen said, "My secret is to see myself as a person who makes exercise a part of her daily routine. It is a non-negotiable appointment. No matter how I feel, I always put my tennis shoes on. I tell myself that once I get started, if I don't really want to do it, I can stop. Usually, once my heart starts pumping, I feel better and complete some type of workout. I just tailor it to how I feel."

Exercise: Mindful Yoga

There are many beautiful ways to enhance your sense of embodiment through mindful movement. One of my favorite activities is yoga, which, practiced mindfully, can be a healing practice for anyone. I teach it to people of all ages and levels of flexibility. I like to say that if you can breathe, you can do yoga.

Mindful yoga is about being aware of your body and breath while you gently stretch and strengthen it in ways that feel delicious. While the practice is physical in nature, it also helps you calm your mind by continually bringing your attention back to the sensations of your body. Since your mind can only focus on one thing at a time, when you are focused on the body you cannot be focused on your worries, anxieties, fears, angers, and disappointments.

There are many styles of yoga that require different levels of physical ability. So, before you take a new yoga class, it is important to do your research. Regardless of the style, in the west, yoga can turn into a yoga competition instead of a yoga practice. The kind of yoga that I am recommending is one that honors your body and feels supportive and healing. I am a Kripalu-trained teacher, but I know there are other traditions that are lovely as well. One suggestion is to beware of teachers who encourage you to push beyond your limits or comfort zone.

To get started, please visit the New Harbinger website at http://www.newharbinger.com/33278 or my website at http://www.lynnrossy.com and download the videos for any of the three yoga series. Two of them have chair versions you can use if getting on the floor is not possible or desired. One of them has simple standing postures that can be done in almost any outfit. The three things to remember when you're doing yoga are to bring your attention to your breath and your body, do your version of the posture, and be kind and gentle throughout the practice. This will ensure a supportive experience you can enjoy and savor.

CHALLENGES:

- You may have some resistance to paying attention to your body, particularly if you and your body haven't exactly been friends for some time.

- If you typically avoid your body, you are not hearing or heeding its needs for movement.

- Just the word "exercise" can conjure up unpleasant images and feelings.

- Common reasons for not exercising are the lack of time or funds for formal memberships or classes, insufficient energy, and not knowing what to do.

THE GOOD NEWS:

- Overcoming resistance to exercise can be as simple as redefining what it means to you and deciding not to listen to thoughts or beliefs that keep you stuck on the couch.

- An instrumental view of the body helps you appreciate its amazing gifts and treat it well.

- Every movement counts toward preventing chronic diseases produced by a sedentary lifestyle.

- Simply visualizing yourself as an active person can help you become one.

- Valuing the intrinsic aspects of exercise has been shown to positively predict physical self-worth, self-reported exercise behavior, and psychological well-being.

WHAT YOU CAN DO NOW:

- Make Your Plan: Choose an activity you can enjoy, put it on your calendar, be consistent, and visualize yourself as an active person.

- Find ways to move your body throughout the day.

- Thank your body regularly for the daily functions it performs.

- Mindful Yoga: Practice with your own routine or use the recordings on the website. Find the postures that feel best to you and incorporate them into a regular, daily routine.

CHAPTER 8

Making "Healthy Fast Food" in a Hurry-Up World

The world is radically busy and there is a lot of cheap food conveniently available in the drive-through lane and at your local supermarket. You might believe that healthy eating is not affordable and that you don't have time to cook at home. While this might seem true at first glance, if you explore a little bit deeper, you will find plenty of reasons why you can't afford *not to* eat healthy food and make cooking one of your new non-negotiable priorities.

This chapter will help you overcome the barriers to cooking at home and highlight the benefits of sitting down at your own table to eat most of your meals. Just a few simple strategies can help you make friends with your kitchen and discover ways to eat "healthy fast food"—a cooked-at-home meal that's easy, fast, and tasty. If you're a gourmet cook and want to make a more complicated meal, that's great, and I hope you invite me over for dinner. However, for those who think the daily meal is daunting, my motto is "it has to be simple." Simple food made in minutes is the way to healthier eating in a fast-paced world. Learn creative ways to rethink the difficulties, and you might even find yourself having fun in the process.

Finally, experience the joy that mindfulness brings to cooking. There is a beautiful aliveness in your relationship to food that is just waiting to be discovered as you see, smell, feel, and taste the food you transform for your dining pleasure.

THE PERILS OF CONVENIENCE EATING

Apparently a lot of people have bought the message that food should be fast, cheap, and completely convenient. Not only has there been a distinct increase in eating out since 1960, but people spend less time in food preparation even when they eat at home. With the advent of the microwave oven and the associated packaged dinners came the promise to help a growing group of working mothers get food to the table fast. According to a 2010 Harris poll, a little over one half of the people who grew up with home cooking (those 65 or older) cook at home five or more times a week, but only one third of younger Americans report cooking at home regularly (Harris Poll 2010). More shocking is the report that 19 percent of meals consumed every day in the United States are eaten in a car (Pollan 2006)!

Eating out makes eating mindfully and healthfully especially difficult. When you eat out, you tend to be served enormous serving sizes laden with extra calories in the form of extra fat and sugar. You have a hard time finding fresh fruits and vegetables or whole grains. The quality of the food is often questionable and the nutritional value low. The problematic end result is that the common American diet is nutrient poor, with less than 20 percent of meals meeting the United States Department of Agriculture (USDA) guidelines for a healthy diet (Smith, Ng, and Popkin 2013). Further, data indicates that eating out results in people eating more food and more higher-calorie food than people who eat at home, and it shows on the bathroom scale. The more you eat out, the more likely you are to be an unhealthy weight (Kruger, Blanck, and Gillespie 2008).

Unsurprisingly, lack of time is reported as a major barrier to preparing nutritious meals at home, prompting people to "buy" time through the purchase of processed convenience foods and fast food. The tendency to snack throughout the day also decreases time spent cooking, as people reach for portable prepackaged snacks instead of eating meals. Other reasons for eating out include feeling too tired to cook, not knowing what to cook, not knowing how to cook, and being single and living alone.

The common related beliefs that (a) eating healthy is not affordable and (b) eating fast food is cheaper than eating healthy food are important to consider. There are a number of ways to counter these beliefs. My first response is you can't afford *not* to eat healthy. Blatantly obvious is the fact that convenience food is ruining people's health, and we need to find a better way of feeding ourselves on a regular basis. When you eat food that has little nutritional value and high fat and sugar content (as is the case with most convenience food), you will suffer, both from the physical problems that ensue and the medical bills you'll eventually have to pay. My second response is when you eat healthy food, you don't need as much because your body is content with less when your nutritional needs are met and your taste buds are satisfied.

EXTRA BENEFITS OF COOKING AT HOME

Besides being good for your physical health, eating at home can improve your emotional and social well-being. Cooking and eating at home can be a way to bring family and friends together more often. Your social connections improve when you take time for them, and sharing a meal (especially with the TV and phones turned off) creates time every day that's tailor made for connection.

If you have children, eating together at home as a family can provide even further benefits. Many valuable lessons can be taught in the kitchen and around the dinner table. Not only did I sit down to a home cooked meal almost every day of my youth, but the food was often from the backyard garden. This experience trained my taste buds to recognize healthy food and taught me how to prepare it.

If you want your children to consume more healthy food, research indicates you should model eating fruits and vegetables, eat at the table instead of in front of the TV, try unfamiliar foods, don't diet, don't make children clean their plates, and eat more meals together as a family (Patrick and Nicklas 2005). To that I would add—make it fun and creative. Let your children be playful in the kitchen by adding healthy toppings to food, using a variety of colors, decorating your pizza crusts, using cookie cutters to make funny shapes with the food, and blending smoothies together.

"HEALTHY FAST FOOD" DEFINED

To help you get started with healthy eating, whether you have a tight budget or tight time restrictions, I developed the concept of "healthy fast food," complete with strategies for making it happen. This is a guide for cooking simple and fast meals without giving up on health or taste. "Healthy fast food" is food you cook at home that has the following qualities:

1. Easy to cook

2. Fast to prepare (approximately thirty minutes to one hour start to finish)

3. Doesn't break your budget

4. Tastes yummy

5. Good for your body's health

6. Includes ingredients that are organic, local, or seasonal (when possible and recommended)

Let's take a look at these descriptions one at a time.

Easy to Cook

Food is easier to cook if you have basic equipment and basic ingredients on hand. Basic equipment would be a soup/pasta pot, skillet, medium saucepan, baking sheet, casserole dish, three knives (chef's, serrated bread, and paring), and a vegetable peeler. My kitchen basics include the following:

In the Cupboard

Salt and black pepper

Spices and herbs of your choosing

Extra-virgin olive oil

Sherry or wine vinegar

Balsamic vinegar

Soy sauce

Hot sauce and barbecue sauce

Pasta, rice, noodles, and grains

Canned beans

Canned tomatoes and tomato paste

Nut butter of your choosing

Nuts and seeds

In the Fridge

Fresh vegetables and greens in season—LOTS!

Fresh fruit in season

Milk, butter, and yogurt

Eggs

Cheese, including good Parmesan cheese

Mustard and ketchup

Onions

Potatoes

Ginger

Lemons and/or limes

Bacon

Pickles, olives, and capers

Salsa

In the Freezer

Frozen vegetables

Frozen fruit

Soup stocks

Pesto

Tomato sauce

Leftover vegetables to put in stock

Meats to thaw or put in crockpot

Of course, this is a list of bare basics and you always need to add your favorites. For instance, I always have a tub of hummus or guacamole and blue corn chips to snack on when I come home way too hungry to wait for dinner. If I do that, a salad usually suffices for dinner. Depending on your style of eating (e.g., vegan, vegetarian) or medical condition (e.g., food allergies or sensitivities), you will alter your list accordingly.

Making it easy also means redefining what "dinner" means. Dinner doesn't have to mean a three-course meal or complex dishes. Some of my favorite simple dinners are a baked sweet potato with black beans, cheese, and salsa on top; roasted chicken with a salad; a large salad with meat, beans, or nuts added for protein; soup with bread and cheese; an egg omelet with vegetables; and pizza with any kind of topping. For Sunday dinner my family has a tradition of eating popcorn, good cheese, nuts, and apples. That's it! Dinner is served.

Fast to Prepare

Along with redefining what constitutes a meal, a couple of other things make dinner fast to prepare—planning ahead and asking for help. Plan ahead by deciding what you're going to cook each night, and make a list of the ingredients that you'll need. Do your grocery shopping for the week at one time. You will be ready to step into the kitchen and get started.

Asking for help from the people you live with—young and old, male or female—can speed up the process of cooking. As I mentioned earlier, cooking together can be important family time and helps you catch up with each other from the day. It also teaches children good habits to take into their adult lives.

Doesn't Break Your Budget

There are a number of ways to stay within your budget when you feed yourself. You can buy generic brands or store brands, stock up on nonperishables when they go on sale, buy in bulk, go meatless a few days a week, shop for vegetables and fruits in season, and buy fruits and vegetables by the bag instead of individually. You can grow a garden in the summer and freeze what you don't use to cook throughout the winter. You can save a ton of money by eating breakfast at home, taking your own snacks and lunch, and making coffee at home to take to work in a thermal mug. According to the Accounting Principals (2013) Workonomixs Survey, the average American worker spends about $36 a week on lunch and more than $20 a week on coffee.

With that said, I do have certain ingredients that I spend a little extra on because of the bang I get for my buck. I will definitely splurge on aged balsamic vinegar because it literally transforms a salad into something spectacular. I have people comment all of the time about how good my salads are and the secret ingredient is the best balsamic vinegar I can afford. I also splurge on cheese. I shop at a local store that imports cheeses from around the world. While the cheese isn't local, at least the store is. There is hardly anything better than a good parmigiano reggiano, and it's essential for the pesto I make in the summer. Decide for yourself what you can pay less for and what you will buy at a higher price. Let your taste buds and your pocketbook decide. If you can't afford higher quality ingredients, it's still better to cook at home with what you can afford.

Tastes Yummy

When you eat mindfully (using the BASICS of mindful eating), it is very difficult to eat food that doesn't taste yummy. Through the process of paying attention and being present to taste, your body will guide you to eat what you can savor. You might be surprised by what you hear. On a regular basis, I have people tell me they discover something new about what they do and do not like. Very simple foods can taste yummy, particularly when they are fresh, local, and in season. The forbidden foods that you thought you liked might be distasteful to you. Stay tuned every time you eat and notice if what you enjoy changes over time. Don't settle for food you don't like.

Good for Your Body's Health

To a large degree, your body and taste buds will guide you to eat in a way that supports greater health. Each time you eat, pay attention mindfully to how your body responds to different food and then behave accordingly. So, if you notice that you feel terrible after eating something (like when I eat French fries), then you may want to eliminate or reduce the times that you eat that food. I still eat French fries occasionally, but only healthy versions baked in the oven.

Besides listening to your body, it can be helpful to know a little about foods that are thought to be particularly good for you and, if you like them, add them to your basic list of ingredients. According to Elaine Magee (2010), super foods boost your intake of vitamins, minerals, and other key nutrients that the body needs to be healthy. Super foods include grapes (purple, red, and blue), blueberries, red berries (especially strawberries and raspberries), nuts (many different kinds), dark green veggies (e.g., broccoli, spinach, kale, and collard greens), sweet potatoes and other orange vegetables (e.g., carrots and squash), tea (particularly green), whole grains, beans, and fish.

NutritionAction.com is a newsletter published by the nonprofit Center for Science in the Public Interest (CSPI), a consumer advocacy organization that regularly reviews the latest research findings on nutrition and health. Its booklet, *Healthy Foods: Your Guide to the*

Best Basic Foods (Lieberman and Hurley 2012), provides a list of the top ten recommended foods: sweet potatoes, mangoes, unsweetened Greek yogurt, broccoli, wild salmon, crispbreads, garbanzo beans, watermelon, butternut squash, and leafy greens.

An even simpler way to remember how to eat is by looking for variety and color. Each color represents different nutrients found in food. For instance, red and orange fruits and vegetables are high in vitamin C, orange and yellow foods are high in carotenoids that create vitamin A, green vegetables are high in iron, and blue and purple foods are high in antioxidants. It's easy to get into a habit of eating the same thing over and over again. Branching out and eating a rainbow of colors and variety of foods can make dinner more interesting, pleasurable, and nutritious.

Organic, Local, or Seasonal Ingredients

At the risk of sounding elitist, when I use ingredients that are organic, local, or seasonal, I am more likely to enjoy the taste and my body feels better eating it. I know that budgets and time can make eating this way challenging, but there is some evidence that it is better for your health, and I think it is worth moving in that direction as much as your pocketbook and schedule will allow. I will go into more of the reasons why in the next chapter, but here are a couple of highlights.

With regard to organic food, there are conflicting results in the scientific literature. Two large systematic reviews looked at the differences between organic and nonorganic food. The first study was conducted by researchers at Stanford University who compiled evidence from 237 peer-reviewed publications. They concluded there is little nutritional difference between organic and conventional food but report that organic foods have significantly less pesticides, synthetic fertilizers, hormones, and antibiotics (Smith-Spangler et al.

2012). The second study was conducted by researchers from Europe and the United States and compiled evidence from 343 peer-reviewed publications. This meta-analytic study revealed that organic crops and crop-based foods are significantly higher in anti-oxidants, lower in the toxic metal cadmium, and lower in pesticide residues than nonorganic (Baranski et al. 2014).

With that said, certain foods are more important to buy organic than others. The Environmental Working Group, a nonprofit organization, provides buyer's guides based on USDA tests of pesticide residues found on food products. Their "Dirty Dozen" list of foods highest in pesticide loads in 2015 consists of apples, peaches, nectarines, strawberries, grapes, celery, spinach, sweet bell peppers, cucumbers, cherry tomatoes, imported snap peas, and potatoes. In addition, if leafy greens and hot peppers are eaten frequently, they recommend that they be organically grown because of the highly toxic chemicals that can be found on them. On the other hand, their "Clean Fifteen" list of produce least likely to hold pesticide residues consists of avocados, sweet corn, pineapples, cabbage, frozen sweet peas, onions, asparagus, mangoes, papaya, kiwis, eggplant, grapefruit, cantaloupe, cauliflower, and sweet potatoes.

Eating organic food is especially important for children and for women who are pregnant or breast-feeding. However, if it is good for developing brains and bodies, a lot of people apparently believe it could be could for them too. According to a survey by the Organic Trade Association (2015a), sales of organic food and non-food products have been rising steadily—11.3 percent in the past year. In another survey, 78 percent of organic food buyers said they typically buy their organic foods at conventional food stores or supermarkets (Organic Trade Association 2015b). Fortunately, as many large food chains have started to see the value in selling organic produce, the result is that more of it is being produced—lowering the price at the checkout counter.

Organic or not, food that's produced locally and food that's in season will be fresher and taste better. Your local farmers market or Community Supported Agriculture (CSA) can help make local, seasonal produce accessible year round. Get to know the farmers who grow your food. Make an outing to the farmers market a family event. The taste of food that's fresh from the farm might turn even the most finicky child into a vegetable eater. Better still, many farmers markets accept food stamps to make organic, local, and seasonable produce available to everyone.

Exercise: The Joy of Mindful Cooking

Take a deep breath and relax your body from head to toe. Imagine yourself smiling in the kitchen, cooking a delicious, healthy, affordable meal. If you imagine yourself cooking with ease, you are more likely to make it happen than if you imagine yourself incapable of the task or impatient with the process. The image of yourself cooking can be flavored with the good feelings that you'll have when you dine on food that you can trust is nurturing you, your friends, and your family.

This week, plan a meal you'd like to cook based on the recommendations in this chapter for "healthy fast food." The key instruction is to take mindful, kind, curious attention into the kitchen. Use mindfulness to help you relax and bring a loving presence to the food. As my French friend (and amazing cook) says, the most special ingredient of any meal is love. It's an ingredient not to forget.

You can start being mindful when you buy the food for your meal. Be aware of where the food comes from, the earth it was grown in, and the sun and rain that stimulated the food to grow. In the kitchen, be aware of the food with all of your senses—see, smell, and touch the food with complete attention. If the mood of the day has followed you into the kitchen and it's a bit sour, just allow it to be there with you as you gather your awareness back to the process of cooking the food and preparing it in a loving way. Just like in sitting meditation practice, when your mind wanders away to something else, gently but firmly and lovingly bring your attention back to all of the senses available to you in the kitchen.

If there are other people at home, ask for their help in preparing the food or the table. Make the table appealing with a tablecloth or placements, nice napkins, a lit candle, and even some flowers. Arrange the food so that it adds to the ambience of the table. Use your good plates instead of waiting for company to treat yourself. You don't have to do these things every day, but pick a day each week to make a beautiful table and see what a difference it makes to the eating experience.

Before you eat, take a moment to be thankful for the food and grateful for the ability to nourish your body. Give yourself a pat on the back for taking the time to prepare this meal for yourself. Eat mindfully and savor every bite.

After the meal, mindfully clean the dishes and the kitchen. Gather your attention to the methodical task of washing, drying, and cleaning. Let thoughts of gratitude fill your mind for the food that nourished you and the kitchen that served you to bring sustenance into your life. The habit of making "healthy fast food" at home is being fortified every time you step into the kitchen and prioritize your health over convenience.

CHALLENGES:

- The world is radically busy, and there is a lot of cheap food conveniently available in the drive-through lane and at your local supermarket.

- Lack of time, feeling too tired to cook, not knowing what to cook, not knowing how to cook, and being single and living alone are barriers to preparing nutritious meals at home.

- Eating out makes eating mindfully and healthfully especially difficult because of enormous serving sizes, extra fat and sugar, lack of fresh fruits and vegetables or whole grains, and the low nutritional value of food.

- Common beliefs that (a) eating healthily is not affordable and (b) eating fast food is cheaper than eating healthy food keep many people from eating healthily.

THE GOOD NEWS:

- Just a few simple strategies can help you make friends with your kitchen and discover ways to eat "healthy fast food"—a cooked-at-home meal that's fast and easy.

- Food is easier to cook if you have some basic ingredients on hand.

- Redefining what constitutes dinner, planning ahead, and asking for help can make "healthy fast food" a reality on a regular basis.

- Healthy food is getting more affordable and you don't have to break the bank to eat organic, local, and seasonal food.

WHAT YOU CAN DO NOW:

- Prepare your kitchen with the basics that you will need to cook fast and easily.

- Make a list of what you will make for dinner for the week and buy the groceries you need.

- Explore farmers markets, CSAs, and other local distributors in your area.

- Make cooking at home a non-negotiable priority as you learn to plan, cook, and eat in ways that are supportive of your health.

- Discover the joy of mindful cooking as you prepare "healthy fast food" for yourself and your friends and family.

CHAPTER 9

Enjoy Every Bite: How to Become a Conscious Connoisseur

Now that you're getting into the mindset of cooking healthy fast food, it's time to take your exploration of food a little bit further. Examining the larger landscape of food production, food quality, and food culture reveals how the choices you make about what to eat not only affect your body but touch the world for better or worse.

Becoming a *conscious connoisseur* will help you develop a passion for both eating delicious food and eating food that contributes to your health, the welfare of others, and the environment. Eating tasty food that's healthy for all is not just an optimistic viewpoint but a truth that can be uncovered as you question how your food choices reflect your personal, social, environmental, political, and spiritual values.

This chapter will encourage you to accept your part in shaping the future of food as you mindfully define your values in regard to it. You will learn that the ability to savor your food is an important step toward savoring your entire life.

WHAT IS A CONSCIOUS CONNOISSEUR?

Food is a wonderful part of our lives and we can enjoy every bite. Being conscious with all aspects of food and being a connoisseur of food can simultaneously increase the pleasure and the health benefits you gain while living in alignment with the world. This is a holistic approach for eating with the fullest pleasure. As author Wendell Berry (2009, 234) said, "Eating with the fullest pleasure—pleasure, that is, that does not depend on ignorance—is perhaps the profoundest enactment of our connection with the world." Becoming a *conscious connoisseur* requires understanding food, pleasure, health, and your role as a human being in a broad context. Let's take each point one at a time.

Being *conscious* with food means

1. being mindful about what, when, why, and how you eat;

2. being a knowledgeable consumer of food so that what and how you eat honors your body and your taste buds; and

3. being conscientious about how your food choices affect the community, the environment, and the world.

Being *a connoisseur* of food means

1. taking time to choose food you really like and food that will satisfy you;

2. being fully present for the experience of eating and taking pleasure in that experience; and

3. exploring the world of food to discover the many varieties of flavors and tastes that are available to enjoy.

BECOMING CONSCIOUS WITH FOOD

Unconscious choices due to mindlessness are not as healthy as the choices you make when you are awake to your actions in each moment. Mindfulness helps you notice the dissonance between unhealthful actions and your ever-growing friendship with your body and connection to the world around you. Being conscious not only improves the direct eating experience but has consequences far beyond the table.

What, When, Why, and How You Eat

Practicing with the BASICS of mindful eating brings consciousness to what, when, why, and how you eat. It's impossible to follow them perfectly, but every time you eat is an opportunity to awaken to the food you eat. There is no magic involved, just consistent effort to be present and observe. For a review, the BASICS are:

B—Breathe and belly check for hunger and satiety before you eat

A—Assess your food

S—Slow down

I—Investigate your hunger throughout the meal, particularly halfway through

C—Chew your food thoroughly

S—Savor your food

Thankfully, you will find that you do not have to sacrifice taste in order to eat food that's good for your body. After exploring the concept of a *conscious connoisseur* for a few weeks, Amy said there was a "conscious recognition that the previously craved foods full of sugar and fat were cheap in quality, not that pleasurable, and not worth eating." Eating mindfully can feel like a celebration of your body's wisdom.

Honor Your Body and Your Taste Buds

Foods with sugar, fat, and salt exert an amazing pull on you if you don't use mindfulness to eat them responsibly. Sugar and fat are needed to give the body energy, and salt is an essential nutrient. You don't have to completely avoid sugar, fat, or salt. But, being conscious of how you feel when you eat food with these ingredients can give you the information you need about what, when, and how much to consume.

When you eat without shame or guilt—free of old beliefs about what you should and should not eat—the results might surprise you. Even though Sally had started taking her lunch to work, she still liked "the idea" of having a cheeseburger and French fries with a soda for lunch (it was an old tape). Despite that thought, Sally was pleased at how delightful the carrots, apple, a simple sandwich, and water were that she packed for lunch. In addition, she was satisfied well past the midafternoon slump she would have experienced after the burger meal.

As Sally discovered, what you eat affects how you feel, the energy you have, and how satisfied you are after you eat. Your body is waiting for you to listen and respond. When you slow down and pay attention, you can hear the internal voice of health surface from beneath the clamor of other conditioned voices. By knowing which types of food bring the body into greater balance, you will be less likely to overeat, and eating will begin to feel like a loving act instead of a guilt-producing activity.

The basic idea is to eat food you enjoy that nutritionally has staying power. In general, these are foods that are unpackaged and unprocessed. You might call it *real food* rather than *food-like substances*, as Michael Pollan would say. In his book *In Defense of Food*, Pollan (2008) suggests avoiding food products containing ingredients that (a) are unfamiliar, (b) are unpronounceable, (c) number more than five, or (d) include high fructose corn syrup. While none of these characteristics is necessarily harmful in and of itself, they are all reliable markers for foods that have been highly processed. Quite simply, food that is closer to its source will supply more energy for your body.

Please notice any tendency to turn these suggestions into rules for yourself that you feel guilty about breaking. There will be times you will eat past the point of satiety or eat something that is considered unhealthy. That's okay. The key is to be conscious about your choices and realize this journey is about progress, not perfection. It is what you eat over the long term that makes a difference. Each time you choose food that honors your body and your taste buds, you will be building a repertoire of experiences that bring a sense of well-being to your body and heart.

The Impact of Your Food Choices

Knowledge about the far-reaching impact of your food choices can be both disheartening and empowering. While you might not pause to consider it very often, how you eat plays a big role in determining what food is produced, how it is produced, the size of the carbon footprint, our water quality, and the health of our ecosystems. While most of us weren't paying attention, many food systems (production, processing, packaging, transportation, distribution) have had serious negative impacts on the quality of our food and the environment. It can be a little shocking to wake up to the results of our processed, fast food culture.

One of the movements trying to counteract the negative impact of the toxic food environment is the Slow Food movement, started in the 1980s by a group of activists led by Carlo Petrini in Italy. Their demonstration against the proposal to build a McDonalds at the Spanish Steps in Rome has turned into an international movement. The initial aim was to defend regional traditions, good food, gastronomic pleasure, and a slow pace of life. It has evolved into a global movement involving thousands of projects and millions of people in over 160 countries.

The philosophy of the Slow Food movement rests on three principles: good, clean, and fair. In other words, it promotes food that is of good quality, flavorsome, and healthy; it encourages clean food production that does not harm the environment; and it supports fair, accessible prices for consumers and fair conditions and pay for producers. While these might sound like lofty ideals, having a vision about what you want your world to look like is an essential place to start.

The good news is that you *can* make a difference by making small changes in what you buy and eat. Here is a list of suggestions that can help you be a conscious consumer of food:

- *Go meatless one day a week*—"Meatless Monday" began in 2003 in association with the Johns Hopkins Bloomberg School of Public Health. According to the Meatless Monday website, "skipping meat one day a week is good for you, great for your nation's health, and fantastic for the planet" (Monday Campaigns, Inc. 2015). The website has lots of recipes to bring meatless magic to your dinner table. Eating less meat may reduce your risk of a number of chronic and preventable diseases, reduce your carbon footprint, and save resources such as fossil fuels and fresh water. In fact, the Natural Resources Defense Council (2010) estimates that if all Americans eliminated just one quarter-pound serving of beef per week, the reduction in global warming gas emissions would be equivalent to taking four to six million cars off the road!

- *Buy local food*—There are many ways to buy local these days, even in small towns. You can go to the farmers market or shop at the grocery stores in your area that sell food from local producers. Eating local reduces your carbon footprint by minimizing emissions caused by transportation of goods.

- *Grow your own food*—You can't get more local than your backyard. Not only does it feel good to harvest your own food for the dinner table, but the taste is definitely going to win you over. There are many resources on the web and probably in your local community for learning how to get started with your first vegetable garden.

- *Use all of your food*—I know I've told you to throw food away that your body isn't hungry for, but there are a number of other choices to consider. You can cook only what you'll eat, eat what's left over the next day, or compost the food you don't eat. Composting food scraps will provide you with rich, nutrient-dense soil for growing your food or enhancing your flowerbeds. For more suggestions, go to http://www.thinkeatsave.org. This organization is dedicated to conscious consumption and teaching people how to have a smarter relationship with food—how we eat it, serve it, shop for it, and dispose of it. Estimates indicate Americans waste one third to one half of all of the food that's produced, so we have a lot of room to improve.

- *Eat whole foods*—Whole foods don't have as much of an impact on the environment as food that's been refined and processed. Whole grains, for example, not only minimize factory usage but enhance your energy level by keeping your blood sugar levels stable, help lower cholesterol, help prevent the formation of small blood clots that can trigger heart attacks or strokes, and may protect against some cancers (Harvard T.H. Chan School of Public Health 2015).

As an individual consumer, your decisions about what food to eat shape your body, the bodies of those around you, the degree to which the earth is treated in a sustainable way, the extent to which industry controls the marketplace, and how connected you feel to the nature sustaining you. Wendell Berry (2009, 231) states that eating "is inescapably an agricultural act, and that how we eat determines, to a considerable extent, how the world is used." Because of your intimate connection to the world, every bite of food you take makes a statement about your personal, social, environmental, political, and spiritual values. You can consciously eat and live by *your* values, not the values set by corporate agriculture.

BECOMING A CONNOISSEUR

I love food and I love to eat good food, so helping others feel the same way gives me great pleasure. Unfortunately, food can be seen as an enemy and a necessary evil to be dealt with on a daily basis. By becoming a connoisseur—a discerning, appreciative consumer of food—any displeasure with eating can be transformed into an act of love, delight, beauty, and art.

Choosing Delicious, Satisfying Food

I often get some giggles when I tell people to eat delicious food. I am told, "That's the problem. When food is really delicious I can't stop myself from eating too much." However, the opposite can be true. When you take time to choose and prepare food in a way that pleases your sense of smell, sight, and taste, you can experience a sense of satisfaction without overeating. The focus is on quality, not quantity. Giving yourself the quality that you desire can lead to a decrease in the quantity of food that you eat, because you are satisfied sooner.

How many times have you grazed throughout the kitchen eating everything in sight except the one thing you really wanted, only to finally have what you wanted in the first place? Giving yourself what you want first can keep you from eating lots of unnecessary food. When you eat what you really want, in an environment without guilt, you will be able to discern what your taste buds really enjoy.

Caitlin had been practicing mindful eating for a few weeks when she found herself craving foods she had previously forbidden. She let herself have what she wanted but discovered that the ingredients were cheap in quality and the taste was equally cut-rate. Her conscious recognition that the craved foods weren't all that pleasurable made it easy for her not to eat them again. It gave her a sense of relief to let them go and embrace the quality of food that brought more lasting pleasure.

Shirley noticed through the practice of mindful eating that she was getting pickier about what she ate. She admitted to herself she didn't really like cheap chocolate or cheap peanut butter. She began slowly savoring quality chocolate and consumed much less. She started grinding her own almond butter. She noticed that processed food leaves an unpleasant aftertaste and doesn't offer the flavor and satisfaction that whole foods provide.

Be Fully Present for the Pleasure of Eating

Of course, the only way to know what you find delicious and satisfying is to be fully present for the experience of tasting, seeing, and smelling. Consciously tuning in to your senses each time you eat will strengthen your inner connoisseur. Ask yourself, *Is this food I can savor? Is this food pleasing to the eye and a pleasure to smell? Does this food bring me to life or drag me down? Does this food feel supportive to my well-being on every level?*

Eating this way can begin to turn every eating experience into a pleasurable one. This doesn't mean you have to eat a gourmet meal every time you sit down. Even eating simple foods—a piece of fresh fruit, for instance—can provide a satisfying, delightful experience.

The art of eating as a connoisseur requires your presence at the table. Make the experience one of beauty whenever you can. Bring out the good dishes or eat in a beautiful natural environment. Put on some dinner music. Buy some flowers to put on the table. You are worth it, and you deserve to have beauty in your life.

Explore the Wonderful World of Food

As you cultivate your senses through mindful observation, don't be surprised if you become dissatisfied with some of your usual food choices. Use this as an exciting opportunity to explore the wonderful world of food. Here are a few suggestions to help you get started:

- *Spice up your life.* Try different kinds of spices found in cultures around the world. Each country has a variety of cuisines—each distinct region having utilized what's best and available. Dive into a country of your choice and see how your taste buds come alive with each new spicy experience.

- *Use cookbooks, food blogs, and recipe websites.* With the explosion of interest in food, you have no excuse for eating the same thing every day. You can type ingredients available in your kitchen into your search engine and see pages of recipe suggestions.

- *Introduce new and unfamiliar fruits and vegetables.* When I lived in Mexico for four months, I was amazed at the fruits and vegetables I had never seen or tasted. Even in my own country, I discovered new vegetables when I subscribed to Community Supported Agriculture (CSA) to purchase produce. The CSA provided recipes for all the food, which made them easy to cook. Farmers markets are a great place to explore for seasonal produce you've never tried before.

- *Try a new restaurant or dish.* Vacations are great times to try new food and food that's special to an area. My vacation pictures are replete with food shots and delectable memories. These outings give me ideas for what to cook when I get back home. When at home, try a restaurant you haven't been to before or try a new dish at a familiar restaurant.

- *Learn from others.* Ask a friend who cooks really well for recipe suggestions or cooking tips. Better yet, take a cooking class. This combines social time with cooking time, and everyone benefits.

- *Shop at ethnic grocery stores.* These are treasure troves of new food experiences. Take some time to prowl the aisles and ask the owner for suggestions on what to try and how to cook a particular type of food.

- *Have a potluck.* Invite a bunch of friends over and ask them to bring copies of the recipe for the dish they make. At one potluck I asked everyone to make something with at least one ingredient from our local international food store. Of course, you can create any theme that you want. The bigger the party, the more new ideas you get.

The success of the food movements is making it easier for you to become a *conscious connoisseur.* Local food movements such as the farm-to-table movement are focused on connecting food producers and food consumers in the same region, reducing the need to buy food from faraway places.

Taking small steps can make a difference, and we can't afford to live in ignorance about the effects of our choices. Endeavor to make more of your eating experiences satisfying and pleasurable, both on an individual and global level. Get playful. Get creative. And discover the joy of eating that goes beyond the taste of the food but includes the pleasure you get from knowing you are contributing to the health of your body, your fellow human beings, and the planet.

Exercise: Choiceless Awareness Meditation

It's time to sit in meditation again so you can let all of this information settle into your heart and mind, to be held lightly with kindness and compassion. This meditation will help you be choicelessly aware of all of your senses from moment to moment. This practice teaches you to be open and accepting of experiences without strain or struggle, setting the stage for insight and wisdom to arise. See if you can experience the truth that all things are constantly changing; and, with this knowledge, see if you can experience the freshness of life—yours and that of the world around you. Each moment is a new beginning and a new opportunity to wake up to the world around you and within you. Do the following exercise for fifteen minutes, if possible, to give yourself the gift of presence. You can download an audio recording of this exercise at http://www.newharbinger.com/33278 or http://www.lynnrossy.com.

> Start by sitting for a few moments as you settle into an erect yet relaxed posture. Let your eyes close or simply lower your gaze to the ground as you take your attention to your body and your breath. Briefly scan the body from head to toe and see if you can soften and release any tension you might find. Take a couple of deep breaths to help you relax and settle into this moment—into your body and into your breath. Settle into the natural rhythm of your breath. No need to control the breath in any way. It might be deep or shallow. Let the breath breathe itself.
>
> Once you feel like your mind has settled, you can let go of the attention on breath and become open and aware of all sensations as they pass through the field of your awareness. Let sensations of sound, touch, taste, smell, sight, and thought naturally arise and fall away. Notice the changing nature of all the senses. Sounds come and go, thoughts come and go, body

sensations pulse and throb and change, the breath changing with each new moment.

Be aware of your experience of being alive without judgment, with kindness and open acceptance. Not resisting anything. Not opposing anything. Notice the whole play of life flowing through you.

If you get caught in your thoughts—a story that grabs your attention—simply notice with a slight smile as you recognize the busy mind and shepherd your attention to rest on the breath for a few moments to stabilize your practice. When you're ready, open back up to all sensations. Letting go of any agenda to make something happen. Letting life be exactly as it is. Resting in presence. Enjoy the sensations of being alive.

CHALLENGES:

- Unconscious choices due to mindlessness are generally not as healthy as the choices you make when you are awake to your actions in each moment.

- Foods with sugar, fat, and salt exert an amazing pull on you if you don't use mindfulness to eat them responsibly.

- When food is really delicious, it can be a challenge to stop yourself from eating too much.

- While most of us weren't paying attention, many food systems have had serious negative impacts on the quality of our food and the environment.

THE GOOD NEWS:

- You do not have to sacrifice taste in order to eat food that's good for your body.

- You *can* make a statement about your values with small changes in what you buy and eat.

- When you take time to choose and prepare food in a way that pleases your sense of smell, sight, and taste, you can experience a sense of satisfaction without overeating.

- By becoming a connoisseur—a discerning, appreciative consumer of food—any displeasure with eating can be transformed into an act of love, delight, beauty, and art.

WHAT YOU CAN DO NOW:

- Pick one idea from this chapter to improve on what you are already doing to live from a place of heart and connection when it comes to food. Be mindfully aware of how this new activity is experienced by all of your senses, how it changes your relationship to yourself and the world, and how it empowers you in the rest of your life. After you feel comfortable with one idea, explore another step as you take the ever-unfolding journey of becoming a *conscious connoisseur*.

CHAPTER 10

Continuing on the Path of Mindful Eating and Living

The end of this book is really the beginning of years of discovery. The lessons of mindful eating and living unfold every moment, day, week, year—your entire lifetime. The only requirement is your loving attention. And, the gift you receive will be whatever you require in the moment—helping you to let go of that which does not serve you and embrace the health, joy, and wisdom that nurtures your well-being.

In this last chapter, major lessons from the book will be highlighted. You will be asked to reflect on what you want to do now to continue your journey of mindful eating and living, what barriers might get in your way, and how you will overcome them. You will be asked to deeply consider a commitment to a regular mindfulness practice.

With a bounty of available resources, I'll share just a few I have found helpful and encourage you to explore others through your own investigations. With the new awareness of your body, heart, and mind, you will notice many things before unseen and be guided in ways you haven't been before.

To end, the practice of gratitude will be offered as a way of honoring who you are right now and the miracle of your life in this moment.

MAJOR LESSONS

Following is a list of ten important takeaways from this book. As you explore them all, notice how your understanding of them deepens over time. Notice and write down others you would like to remember.

1. The switch from a diet mentality to a mindfulness approach will guide you to savor the food you love and love the way you *feel* after you eat, without having more than you need.

2. The practice of formal and informal mindfulness will strengthen your ability to make conscious choices in every area of your life.

3. The BASICS of mindful eating are a complete set of guidelines to help you become conscious about what, when, why, and how you eat. Use them as often as possible when you sit down to eat.

4. The Three Food Wisdoms (eating with permission, eating the "right amount," and knowing and respecting your habits and triggers with food) will help you release the idea of forbidden foods and eat without shame and guilt.

5. Negative thoughts do not need to run your life (they aren't true). Instead, you can cultivate kind and helpful self-talk that inspires you to be your best self.

6. Emotions are natural and normal, mentionable and manageable. They don't have to be reasons to reach for food.

7. What you're really, really, really hungry for is often not food, but a desire for connection, love, creativity, inspiration, silence, rest, and movement.

8. Exercise can be defined as moving your body in ways that feel delicious while appreciating its instrumental value—a true celebration of your body.

9. To eat well on a budget, make "healthy fast food" and take back the kitchen for your health and well-being.

10. Become a *conscious connoisseur* by delighting in food with the fullest pleasure—pleasure that comes from an understanding of the connection between the food you eat, your health, and the health of the planet.

YOUR PERSONAL PLAN OF ACTION

Write down a plan based on what you've learned so far and what you know about the difficulties you've had in the past. Here is what I'd suggest:

1. Write down the top three things you would like to focus on to support mindful eating and living—anything from using the BASICS of mindful eating to exercising.

2. Write down three barriers that might get in your way and the method for overcoming them. For example, if you want to use the BASICS more often when you eat but you often forget, write them down on a card to carry with you, tape them to your refrigerator, or tape them to your computer.

3. Write down a schedule for when you will practice mindfulness every day. This one is so important that I will discuss it in further detail below.

MINDFULNESS MEDITATION PRACTICE

There might be a number of reasons why you think you should skip this section. *I can't meditate because (a) I don't have time, (b) my mind is constantly chattering, (c) sitting doesn't work for me, and (d) I have too many things to do.* Every meditator has had those same thoughts. It doesn't mean you can't meditate or benefit significantly from a mindfulness practice.

Here are some ways to start and keep a meditation practice that can serve you for life:

1. *Choose a time.*

    Try different times to discover what works in your schedule. Long-term meditators often meditate in the morning before their day gets started. That way nothing else gets in the way and the meditation has a positive impact on the rest of the day. But, you need to find the time that works for you. Keep experimenting until you find your rhythm.

2. *Choose a place.*

    I have read recommendations that say "find a quiet place." However, that can be impossible unless you're cloistered in a retreat center somewhere (and even then, you would be surprised at the distractions). Don't let the sounds and activities of your family, pets, phones, TVs, radios, and neighbors make you think you can't meditate at home. Noises are part of life. It can be helpful to minimize them, but if noise is present, you can just use sound as your object of meditation.

    I do think it is helpful to create one place in your home set aside for practice. An energy develops in that location over time that calls you to practice.

3. *Use a timer.*

    If you don't want to sit there the whole time wondering how long it's been, use the timer on your phone or a meditation app to time your meditation sessions. Insight Timer is an app that rings a bell at the end and lets you know how many other people in the world have been meditating with you.

4. *Prepare your body to sit.*

Sitting meditation can be uncomfortable when you first get started because you are not used to sitting still and being quiet. You might discover lots of aches and pains and lots of thoughts you didn't notice before. Relax the body and mind by doing a few stretches before you sit down to meditate.

5. *Be relaxed yet alert.*

Many of us are "stressed and alert" as opposed to "relaxed and alert," which is our ideal condition. You want to be relaxed when you sit but not so relaxed that you fall asleep. You want to be alert without being tense. Take a few deep breaths to wake yourself up and relax you so you can find that sweet spot—not too tense and not too relaxed.

6. *Practice with a slight smile.*

Thich Nhat Hanh suggests bringing a slight smile to your face while you are practicing (and throughout your entire day). A smile sends messages to your brain that you're happy, and the body and mind begin to relax. Here is a short saying you can use from *Peace Is Every Step* (Nhat Hanh 1992, 6): "Breathing in, I calm my body. Breathing out, I smile. Dwelling in the present moment. I know this is a wonderful moment!" Put a smile on your face right now and see how it makes you feel.

7. *Do something every day.*

Set an intention to practice every day. Decide how long you want to sit. While longer sittings (twenty to thirty minutes) will be more beneficial, doing a mini-meditation for two minutes or even five breaths can be enough to center you and bring you back into your life with more clarity and calm. It's more important to do something every day than do nothing at all.

8. *Find support for your practice.*

Meditating with a group of people can support your practice. There are meditation groups at churches, yoga centers, and Buddhist centers that might interest you. In addition, there are many meditation CDs and classes to explore online. Don't forget you can find many meditation recordings on my website at http://www.lynnrossy.com.

9. *Be kind to yourself.*

If you've learned one thing from this book, I hope it is the importance of being kind and gentle with yourself. You are doing the best you can every day and you are amazing for having read this book! Always check to see if you're being kind and gentle to yourself, to your practice, and in your life. Breathe. Soften.

10. *Start over.*

If you forget to practice for a day or even a week, start over. Every day is a new day for recommitting to yourself and to your mindfulness practice. The moment is always available in which to start again. To enjoy the benefits of mindfulness, a regular practice will enrich every aspect of your life.

A TINY RESOURCE LIST

The Center for Mindful Eating (http://www.thecenterformindful eating.org) is a web-based nonprofit organization that offers teleconferences, webinars, and newsletters about every aspect of mindful eating. They have an online bookstore for books on mindful eating and meditation, as well as citations of current research on mindful eating. For professionals, there are continuing education credits available and handouts to use with clients.

For up-to-date, evidence-based diet and nutrition information, go to "The Nutrition Source" on the Harvard T.H. Chan School of Public Health website (http://www.hsph.harvard.edu/nutrition source). It offers information on what's healthy to eat, the latest nutrition news, and home-cooking recipes.

Any cookbook by Mark Bittman will give you lots of bang for your buck. His book *How To Cook Everything Fast* (Bittman 2014) is a solid, worthwhile investment. Many of the recipes fit into my guidelines for "healthy fast food" and, with over 900 pages of recipes, I think you will find enough to keep you busy for a while. He even color codes the recipes to separate tasks between helpers. Other good ones include *Vegetables Every Day* (Bishop 2001), *Vegetarian Cooking for Everyone* (Madison 2007), and *The Very Best Recipes for Health* (Shulman 2010). For anyone on a budget, your local library is the place to try out cookbooks for free.

Food bloggers and apps abound to help you find recipes and eat healthfully within a budget. Do a little exploring to find the ones that appeal to you. I love the New York Times Cooking app, with recipes classified for easy searching; and I love the motto "my stomach is full, and my wallet is too" on the Budget Bytes website (http://www.budgetbytes.com). Recipes on this site even list the dollar amount per serving.

There are many other resources that are equally as good. A simple internet search of key words can help you find them.

THE GIFT OF GRATITUDE

The road of mindful eating is about the journey. It is not about a destination—a place where you can stop and not pay attention anymore. No matter how many times you eat too much and no matter how many times you think you want to give up on yourself, your commitment to the journey will help you get up, brush the dirt off, and start over again.

Don't beat yourself up for not being perfect. (Hint: Nobody's perfect.) Many years ago, I decided to give up seeking perfection. To the perfectionist, nothing is ever good enough, and that mentality sucks the joy out of everything. Instead, I decided to make "imperfection" my goal, and I am happily successful at it every day. Make imperfection your goal and see how much lighter you feel.

So give yourself a break. Embrace and be grateful for your beautiful imperfection. Be grateful for the opportunity to try and learn and grow. Be grateful for the opportunity to fail. Failing is sometimes the best teacher of all. It points you to the lessons you have to learn and the tenderness you need to cultivate in order to face the never-ending ups and downs in life.

Keep working with the suggestions and tips in this book. You will gradually see how the wisdom of mindful eating changes your relationship to food, to your body, and to your life. You may be astonished when you find yourself making better choices with food, eating only what the body needs, and talking to yourself with greater kindness and compassion. Your ability to comprehend what you're really hungry for will grow over time. And your courage to satisfy those hungers will help you truly savor your entire life.

To end, I'd like to offer the following simple meditation on gratitude. Use it on a regular basis and particularly on difficult days to remind your heart and mind of the many blessings that are always available in the here and now. You can download an audio recording of this exercise at http://www.newharbinger.com/33278 or http://www.lynnrossy.com.

Exercise: Gratitude Meditation

Find a comfortable place to rest your body, be relaxed, and gently close your eyes. Let go of any concerns and worries and preoccupations. Allow yourself to be fully present exactly as you are. Nowhere else to go. Nothing else to do.

Allow your attention to rest on the breath at the heart center. Feel the breath moving in and out at the center of the chest. Feel this breath that keeps you alive from moment to moment. Feel the beating of your heart—the heart that generates life throughout your body. Experience this precious gift of being alive. Feel a sense of gratitude for your life and say a soft "thank you."

Scan the body and experience the senses available to you—your eyes can see, your ears can hear, your nose can smell, your mouth can taste, and your body can feel. Consider the blessings these senses offer to your life. Feel gratitude for your body and your health—knowing your body is as healthy as it is capable of being in this moment. Say a soft "thank you" to your body for its gifts.

Bring to mind basic things you normally take for granted—food to eat, water to drink, electricity to light your home, transportation to get you wherever you want to go, and so much more. Say a soft "thank you" to each thing that occurs to you.

Now say a peaceful "thank you" to the beauty of nature, here for your pleasure—the sun, moon, stars, earth, rain, breeze, trees, flowers, and all of the animals, including any pets that you might have.

Bring to mind the people you love and who love you. People you're grateful for, who nourish you and make you laugh. Even bring to mind the people you find challenging—they have gifts to give as well.

Continue for as long as you want as people and circumstances come into your awareness. Feel the gratitude that you have for them. Taking your time. Say a soft "thank you" as each one occurs to you.

Notice what it feels like in the body to feel gratitude. If you're not feeling gratitude, you might be surprised later in the day when something occurs to you. If other thoughts arise, it doesn't matter. When possible, continue to allow things to come to mind that you're grateful for.

See everything in your life as a gift. Be truly grateful for who you are, just as you are, right here and now. You are a miracle and everything around you is a miracle. Know that gratitude is one of the greatest gifts you can give yourself.

And, when you're ready, slowly open your eyes and move into your life with a heart that's filled with blessings.

Acknowledgments

My deepest thanks to all of the people at the University of Missouri and around the world who have taken my classes and had the courage to reexamine their relationship to food and their bodies. Their extraordinary stories of overcoming old beliefs and behaviors to find freedom with food and love of their bodies were my steadfast inspiration while I wrote this book.

Thank you, Laura Schopp, for asking me to develop a class that would help people manage their weight and reduce their health risks. My passion for this work started in that moment. Special thanks to Hannah Bush for using Eat for Life for her dissertation project and to Hannah, Laura, and Laurie Mintz for their help in getting it published.

Thanks to Rick Hanson for his book-writing advice and his referral to Caroline Pincus, who I thank for being my wonderful book midwife.

Thanks to the city of San Francisco for first introducing me to the wonderful world of food. Thanks to the Katy Trail Slow Food Chapter, our local farmers at the Columbia Farmers Market, Sarah and Craig Cyr at Wine Cellar and Bistro, Leigh Lockhart at Main Squeeze, and all of the cookbooks, authors, chefs, friends, and restaurants that have expanded my understanding of taste, food, farm-to-table, sustainability, and the hospitality of the kitchen.

My deepest gratitude to the mindfulness communities that have guided my path for so many years. There are too many teachers, spiritual friends, and organizations to list here, but each one has grounded me in the practice of mindfulness, without which this book would not be possible. And, thanks to New Harbinger for making mindfulness a priority and publishing so many wonderful books on the topic—including mine!

Thanks to all my family and friends who have supported me on this journey—especially Mom and Dad for raising me to love all beings and for modeling service to others; Sarah Swofford for being the best niece and writing co-conspirator; Nancy West for the first thumbs up; Peggy O'Connor, Lara Theriault, and Martha Dragich for their gentle edits; and Althea Harris, Craig Deken, Jan Colbert, Jenny Workman, Katherine Reed, Kim James, Lynn Fair, Melinda Gardner, and Sarah Hill for their love and support through this process.

Finally, thanks to my biggest fan and loving partner, Bud. His ever-present smile reminds me that every day you wake up is a happy one.

References

Accounting Principals. 2013. *Accounting Principals Workonomix Survey 2013*. http://www.accountingprincipals.com/documents /downloads/workonomix_spending_habits.pdf

Agras, W. S., and R. F. Apple. 2007. *Overcoming Your Eating Disorder: A Cognitive-Behavioral Therapy Approach for Bulimia Nervosa and Binge-Eating Disorder*. New York: Oxford University Press.

Andrade, A. M., G. W. Green, and K. J. Melanson. 2008. "Eating Slowly Led to Decreases in Energy Intake Within Meals in Healthy Women." *Journal of the American Dietetic Association* 108(7): 1186–1191.

Baranski, M., D. Srednicka-Tober, N. Volakakis, C. Seal, R. Sanderson, G.B. Stewart, C. Benbrook et al. 2014. "Higher Antioxidant and Lower Cadmium Concentrations and Lower Incidence of Pesticide Residues in Organically Grown Crops: A Systematic Literature Review and Meta-analyses." *British Journal of Nutrition* 112(05): 794–811.

Beck, A. 1967. *Depression: Clinical, Experimental, and Theoretical Aspects*. New York: Hoeber.

Berry, W. 2009. *Bringing It to the Table: On Farming and Food*. Berkeley, CA: Counterpoint.

Bishop, J. 2001. *Vegetables Every Day*. New York: William Morrow Cookbooks.

Bittman, M. 2014. *How to Cook Everything Fast: A Better Way to Cook Great Food.* New York: Houghton Mifflin Harcourt.

Brewer J. A., P. D. Worhunsky, J. R. Gray, Y. Tang, J. Weber, and H. Kober. 2011. "Meditation Experience Is Associated with Difference in Default Mode Network Activity and Connectivity." *Proceedings of the National Academy of Science* 108: 50.

Buettner, D. 2008. *The Blue Zones: Lessons for Living Longer from the People Who've Lived the Longest.* Washington, DC: National Geographic Society.

Burns, D. 1980. *Feeling Good: The New Mood Therapy.* New York: William Morrow.

Bush, H. E., L. Rossy, L. B. Mintz, and L. Schopp. 2014. "Eat for Life: A Worksite Feasibility Study of a Novel Mindfulness-Based Intuitive Eating Intervention." *American Journal of Health Promotion* 28(6): 380–388.

Cameron, J. 2002. *The Artist's Way: A Spiritual Path to Higher Creativity.* New York: Jeremy P. Tarcher/Putnam.

Crum, A. J., and E. J. Langer. 2007. "Mind-Set Matters: Exercise and the Placebo Effect." *Psychological Science* 18(2): 165–71.

Dalen, J., B. W. Smith, B. M. Shelley, A. L. Sloan, L. Leahigh, and D. Begay. 2010. "Pilot Study: Mindful Eating and Living (MEAL): Weight, Eating Behavior, and Psychological Outcomes Associated with a Mindfulness-Based Intervention for People with Obesity." *Complementary Therapies in Medicine* 18(6), 260–264.

Dallman, M. F. 2010. "Stress-Induced Obesity and the Emotional Nervous System." *Trends in Endocrinology and Metabolism* 21(3): 159–165.

De Castro, J. M. 2004. "The Time of Day of Food Intake Influences Overall Intake in Humans." *The American Society for Nutritional Sciences* 134 (1): 104–111.

Domar, A. and H. Dreher. 1996. *Healing Mind, Healthy Woman.* New York: Henry Holt and Company, Inc.

Gast, J. and S. R. Hawks. 2000. "Examining Intuitive Eating as a Weight Loss Program." *Healthy Weight Journal* 14: 42–44.

Gelb, M. 2010. *Wine Drinking for Inspired Thinking: Uncork Your Creative Juices.* Philadelphia, PA: Running Press.

Gleaves, D. H., M. R. Lowe, A. C. Snow, B. A. Green, and K. P. Murphy-Eberenz. 2000. "Continuity in Anorexia Nervosa and Bulimia Nervosa: Co-morbidity and Chronology of Appearance." *Journal of Abnormal Psychology* 109: 56–68.

Goldstein, J. 2003. *Insight Meditation: The Practice of Freedom.* Boston: Shambhala Publications.

Grossman P., L. Niemann, S. Schmidt, and H. Walach. 2004. "Mindfulness-Based Stress Reduction and Health Benefits: A Meta-analysis." *Journal of Psychosomatic Research* 57: 35–43.

Gusella, J., S. Clark, and E. van Roosmalen. 2004. "Body Image Self-Evaluation Colouring Lens: Comparing the Ornamental and Instrumental Views of Adolescent Girls with Eating Disorders." *European Eating Disorders Review* 12(4): 223–229.

Hallowell, E. M. 2005. "Overloaded Circuits: Why Smart People Underperform." *Harvard Business Review* 83(1): 54–62.

Harris Poll. 2010. "Three in Ten Americans Love to Cook, While One in Five Do Not Enjoy It or Don't Cook." http://www.the harrispoll.com/health-and-life/Three_in_Ten_Americans _Love_to_Cook__While_One_in_Five_Do_Not_Enjoy_It _or_Don_t_Cook.html

Harvard T.H. Chan School of Public Health. 2015. "Whole Grains." http://www.hsph.harvard.edu/nutritionsource/whole-grains/

Hawks, S. R., H. Madanat, and A. Harris. 2005. "Relationship Between Intuitive Eating and Health Indicators Among College Women." *American Journal of Health Education* 36(6): 331–336.

Heshmat, S. 2011. *Eating Behavior and Obesity: Behavioral Economics Strategies for Health Professionals.* New York: Springer Publishing Company.

Hong, P. Y., D. A. Lishner, and K. H. Han. 2014. "Mindfulness and Eating: An Experiment Examining the Effect of Mindful Raisin Eating on the Enjoyment of Sampled Food." *Mindfulness* 5(1): 80–87.

Huber, C. 2007. *Making a Change for Good: A Guide to Compassionate Self-Discipline.* Boston: Shambhala.

Joseph, R. J., M. Alonso-Alonso, D. S. Bond, A. Pascual-Leone, and G. L. Blackburn. 2010. "The Neurocognitive Connection Between Physical Activity and Eating Behavior." *Obesity Reviews* 12(10): 800–812.

Kabat-Zinn, J. 1994. *Wherever You Go, There You Are: Mindfulness Meditation in Everyday Life.* New York: Hyperion.

Kabat-Zinn, J. 2013. *Full Catastrophe Living: Using the Wisdom of Your Body and Mind to Face Stress, Pain, and Illness.* New York: Bantam Books.

Katie, B. 2003. *Loving What Is: Four Questions That Can Change Your Life.* New York: Three Rivers Press.

Keng S., M. J. Smoski, and C. J. Robins. 2011. "Effects of Mindfulness on Psychological Health: A Review of Empirical Studies." *Clinical Psychology Review* 31: 1041–1056.

Keys, A., J. Brožek, A. Henschel, O. Mickelsen, and H. L. Taylor. 1950. *The Biology of Human Starvation*. St. Paul: University of Minnesota Press.

Killingsworth, M. A. and D. T. Gilbert. 2010. "A Wandering Mind Is an Unhappy Mind." *Science* 330: 932.

Kimiecik, J. 2009. *The Intrinsic Exerciser: Discovering the Joy of Exercise*. New York: Houghton Mifflin Company.

Kruger, J., H. M. Blanck, and C. Gillespie. 2008. "Dietary Practices, Dining Out Behavior, and Physical Activity Correlates of Weight Loss Maintenance." *Preventing Chronic Disease: Public Health Research, Practice, and Policy* 5:1.

Levine, J. A., M. W. Vander Weg, J. O. Hill, and R. C. Klesges. 2006. "Non-exercise Activity Thermogenesis: The Crouching Tiger Hidden Dragon of Societal Weight Gain." *Arteriosclerosis, Thrombosis, and Vascular Biology* 26(4): 729–36.

Li, J., N. Zhang, L. Hu, Z. Li, R. Li, C. Li, and S. Wang. 2011. "Improvement in Chewing Activity Reduces Energy Intake in One Meal and Modulates Plasma Gut Hormone Concentrations in Obese and Lean Young Chinese Men." *The American Journal of Clinical Nutrition* 94(3): 709–716.

Lieberman, M. D, N. I. Eisenberger, M. J. Crockett, S. M. Tom, J. H. Pfeifer, and B. M. Way. 2007. "Putting Feelings into Words: Affect Labeling Disrupts Amygdala Activity in Response to Affective Stimuli." *Psychological Science* 18(5): 421–428.

Lieberman, M. S. and J. Hurley. 2012. *Healthy Foods: Your Guide to the Best Basic Foods*. Washington, DC: NutritionAction.com

Loehr, J., and T. Schwartz. 2003. *The Power of Full Engagement: Managing Energy, Not Time, Is the Key to High Performance and Personal Renewal*. New York: The Free Press.

Lowe, M. R. and M. L. Butryn. 2007. "Hedonic Hunger: A New Dimension of Appetite?" *Physiology and Behavior* 91: 432–439.

Madison, D. 2007. *Vegetarian Cooking for Everyone.* New York: Broadway Books.

Magee, E. 2010. "10 Nutrient-Rich Super Foods." WebMD. http://webmd.com/food-recipes/10-super-foods

Mann, T., A. J. Tomiyama, E. Westling, A. Lew, B. Samuels, and J. Chatman. 2007. "Medicare's Search for Effective Obesity Treatments: Diets Are Not the Answer." *American Psychologist* 62(3): 220–233.

Marlatt, G. A. and J. Kristeller. 1999. "Mindfulness and Meditation." In *Integrating Spirituality into Treatment: Resources for Practitioners,* edited by W. R. Miller. Washington, DC: American Psychological Association Books.

Merriam-Webster, Inc. 2011. "Biographical Note for Fletcherism." *Medical Dictionary.* http://www.merriam-webster.com/medical/fletcherism

Monday Campaigns, Inc. 2015. "It's Worldwide!" http://www.meatlessmonday.com/the-global-movement/

National Institutes of Health. 2013. "Portion Distortion." https://www.nhlbi.nih.gov/health/educational/wecan/eat-right/portion-distortion.htm

Natural Resources Defense Council. 2010. "Eat Green: Our Everyday Food Choices Affect Global Warming and the Environment." http://www.nrdc.org/globalWarming/files/eatgreenfs_feb2010.pdf

Nhat Hanh, T. 1992. *Peace Is Every Step: The Path of Mindfulness in Everyday Life.* New York: Bantam Books.

Ogden C. L., M. D. Carroll, B. K. Kit, and K. M. Flegal. 2014. "Prevalence of Childhood and Adult Obesity in the United States, 2011–2012." *Journal of the American Medical Association* 311(8): 806–814.

Organic Trade Association. 2015a. *U.S. Organic Industry Survey 2015*. https://www.ota.com/resources/market-analysis

Organic Trade Association. 2015b. *2015 U.S. Families' Organic Attitudes and Beliefs Survey*. https://www.ota.com/resources/market-analysis

Patel, A. V., L. Bernstein, A. Deka, H. S. Feigelson, P. T. Campbell, S. M. Gapstur, G. A. Colditz, and M. J. Thun. 2010. "Leisure Time Spent Sitting in Relation to Total Mortality in a Prospective Cohort of US Adults." *American Journal of Epidemiology* 172(4): 419–429.

Patrick, H. and T. A. Nicklas. 2005. "A Review of Family and Social Determinants of Children's Eating Patterns and Diet Quality." *Journal of the American College of Nutrition* 24: 2, 83–92.

Pedersen, A. M., A. Bardow, S. B. Jensen, and B. Nauntofte. 2002. "Saliva and Gastrointestinal Functions of Taste, Mastication, Swallowing and Digestion." *Oral Diseases* 8(3): 117–129.

Pollan, M. 2004. "Our National Eating Disorder." *The New York Times Magazine*. October 17. http://www.michaelpollan.com/articles-archive/our-national-eating-disorder/

Pollan, M. 2006. *The Omnivore's Dilemma: A Natural History of Four Meals*. New York: Penguin Group.

Pollan, M. 2008. *In Defense of Food: An Eater's Manifesto*. New York: Penguin Press.

Roth, G. 2003. *Breaking Free from Emotional Eating*. New York: Plume.

Ryan, T. 2013. *A Mindful Nation: How a Simple Practice Can Help Us Reduce Stress, Improve Performance, and Recapture the American Spirit*. California: Hay House, Inc.

Sebire, S., M. Standage, and M. Vansteenkiste. 2009. "Examining Intrinsic Versus Extrinsic Exercise Goals: Cognitive, Affective, and Behavioral Outcomes." *Journal of Sport and Exercise Psychology* 31: 189–210.

Shafran, R., B. A. Teachman, S. Kerry, and S. Rachman. 2010. "A Cognitive Distortion Associated with Eating Disorders: Thought-Shape Fusion." *British Journal of Clinical Psychology* 38(2): 167–179.

Shapiro, D. H. 1992. "A Preliminary Study of Long-Term Meditators: Goals, Effects, Religious Orientation, Cognitions." *Journal of Transpersonal Psychology* 24 (1): 23–39.

Shapiro, S. L., L. E. Carlson, J. A. Astin, and B. Freedman. 2006. "Mechanisms of Mindfulness." *Journal of Clinical Psychology* 62: 373–386.

Shulman, M. R. 2010. *The Very Best Recipes for Health: 250 Recipes and More from the Popular Feature on NYTimes.com*. New York: Rodale, Inc.

Smit, H. J., E. K. Kemsley, H. S. Tapp, and J. K. Henry. 2011. "Does Prolonged Chewing Reduce Food Intake? Fletcherism Revisited." *Appetite* 57(1): 295–298.

Smith, L. P., S. W. Ng, and B. M. Popkin. 2013. "Trends in US Home Food Preparation and Consumption: Analysis of National Nutrition Surveys and Time Use Studies from 1965–1966 to 2007–1008." *Nutrition Journal* 12: 45.

Smith, T. and S. R. Hawks. 2006. "Intuitive Eating, Diet Composition, and the Meaning of Food in Healthy Weight Promotion." *American Journal of Health Education* 37: 130–136.

Smith-Spangler, C., M. L. Brandeau, G. E. Hunter, J. C. Bainger, M. Pearson, P. J. Eschbach, V. Sundaram, H. Liu, P. Schirmer, C. Stave, I. Olkin, and D. M. Bravata. 2012. "Are Organic Foods Safer or Healthier than Conventional Alternatives? A Systematic Review." *Annals of Internal Medicine* 157(5): 348–366.

Song, W. O., O. K. Chun, S. Obayashi, S. Cho, and C. E. Chung. 2005. "Is Consumption of Breakfast Associated with Body Mass Index in US Adults?" *Journal of the American Dietetic Association* 105(9): 1373–1382.

Stanchich, L. 1989. *Power Eating Program: You Are How You Eat.* Coconut Grove, FL: Healthy Products, Inc.

Swensen, M. R. 2000. *Say It Again 15,000 Times: Favorite Thoughts and Words of Wisdom.* Anchorage, AK: Publication Consultants.

Tolle, E. 2001. *Practicing the Power of Now: Essential Teachings, Meditation, and Exercises From The Power of Now.* San Francisco: New World Library.

Tolle, E. 2005. *A New Earth: Awakening to Your Life's Purpose.* New York: Dutton/Penguin Group.

Traister, R. 2006. "Getting Over Happiness." *Salon,* February 25, http://www.salon.com/2006/02/25/happiness_4/

Tribole, E. and E. Resch. 1995. *Intuitive Eating: A Revolutionary Program that Works.* New York: St. Martin's Griffin.

Tsafou, K. E., D. T. DeRidder, R. van Ee, and J. P. Lacroix. 2015. "Mindfulness and Satisfaction in Physical Activity: A Cross-Sectional Study in the Dutch Population." *Journal of Health Psychology,* January 28: 1–11.

Tylka, T. L. 2006. "Development and Psychometric Evaluation of a Measure of Intuitive Eating." *Journal of Counseling Psychology* 53(2): 226–240.

Villablanca, P. A., J. R. Alegria, F. Mookadam, D. R. Holmes Jr., R.S. Wright, and J. A. Levine. 2015. "Nonexercise Activity Thermogenesis in Obesity Management." *Mayo Clinic Proceedings* 90(4): 509–19.

Wahlstrom, K. L. and M. S. Begalle. 1999. "More than Test Scores: Results of the Universal School Breakfast Pilot in Minnesota." *Topics in Clinical Nutrition* 15(1): 17–29.

Wansink, B. 2006. *Mindless Eating: Why We Eat More than We Think.* New York: Bantam Books.

Wansink, B. and J. Sobal. 2007. "Mindless Eating: The 200 Daily Decisions We Unknowingly Make." *Environment and Behavior* 39(1): 106–123.

Waters, A., A. Hill, and G. Waller. 2001. "Bulimics' Responses to Food Cravings: Is Binge-Eating a Product of Hunger or Emotional State?" *Behavior Research and Therapy* 39: 877–886.

Wise, J. H. 2002. "The S.T.O.P. Sign Technique." *The Family Journal: Counseling and Therapy for Couples and Families* 10(4): 433–436.

About author

Lynn Rossy, PhD, is a licensed clinical psychologist at the University of Missouri's wellness program for faculty and staff. She developed Eat for Life, a mindfulness-based intuitive eating program that successfully helps people overcome eating issues, improve body image, and enhance weight loss. She is on the board of directors of The Center for Mindful Eating.

MORE BOOKS *from*
NEW HARBINGER PUBLICATIONS

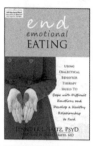
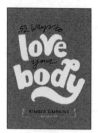
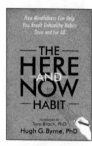
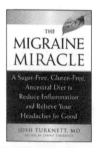
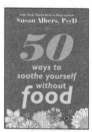
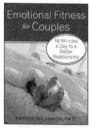